RUN FOREVER

Also by Damian Hall

In It for the Long Run

We Can't Run Away From This

RUN FOREVER

THE SECRETS TO BECOMING AN AGELESS ATHLETE

DAMIAN HALL

WITH RENEE McGREGOR & PETE STABLES

Vertebrate Publishing, Sheffield
www.adventurebooks.com

RUN FOREVER

DAMIAN HALL

First published in 2026 by Vertebrate Publishing. Reprinted in 2026.
VERTEBRATE PUBLISHING, Omega Court, 352 Cemetery Road, Sheffield S11 8FT, United Kingdom.
www.adventurebooks.com

The author has stated to the publishers that, except in such minor respects not affecting the substantial accuracy of the work, the contents of the book are true.

A CIP catalogue record for this book is available from the British Library.

ISBN: 978-1-83981-287-3 (Paperback)
ISBN: 978-1-83981-288-0 (Ebook)
ISBN: 978-1-83981-289-7 (Audiobook)

10 9 8 7 6 5 4 3 2

Vertebrate Publishing is committed to printing on paper from sustainable sources.

FSC www.fsc.org MIX Paper | Supporting responsible forestry FSC® C013604

Printed and bound by CPI Group (UK), Chatham ME5 8TD.

DISCLAIMER
All content within this book is provided for general information only and should not be treated as medical advice. Always consult your doctor or other healthcare professionals if you're in any way concerned about your health.

For Allie

And for everyone determined to grow older disgracefully

CONTENTS

INTRODUCTION
PLAYING THE LONG GAME

'Life's journey is not to arrive at the grave safely, in a well-preserved body, but rather to skid in sideways, totally worn out, shouting, "Holy shit, what a ride!"'

HUNTER S. THOMPSON, GONZO JOURNALIST AND AUTHOR

It's just an average Wednesday morning. But I feel emphatically less than average. I'm breathing like an over-zealous Darth Vader impersonator. My lungs feel like they're tiny Tesco bags. My legs feel like they belong to RoboCop. I'm not doing 400-metre intervals or an uphill tempo. It's meant to be just a standard, zone 1, easy run on the flat. Just a jog, really. But everything about it is more effort than it should be. It feels unusually, puzzlingly, worryingly hard. This easy run is making me feel distinctly uneasy. Something's wrong. And then I remember ...

I did 5 x 3-minute hills yesterday. A tough workout, but one I've done many times. I couldn't still be fatigued from that, could I? Surely not. I'm a runner in my prime. I'm not a professional athlete, but I can just about say, in that singularly British, awkward way, that I'm an elite one. I've represented Great Britain at trail ultramarathon running. I've trained and trained over years and years. I eat chia seeds, get to bed before 11 p.m. and steer well clear of Stella. I have a coach (though I'm also one myself), run six days a week and have barely missed a training run for seven years. I don't want to sound braggy. I'm just explaining that compared to the average population I'm very fit and I don't get tired easily. But here I am, on an average

Wednesday morning, feeling unmistakably and inexplicably below average. I'm doing exactly what I always do. But I'm clearly more tired than usual. Or perhaps, significantly, more tired than I used to get.

Casting aside my invincibility cloak for a moment, didn't I feel like this last week, on my post-workout day, too? And where has my top-end speed been for the last few weeks? Try as I might, I haven't seemed able to quite hit those 5:30 miles I used to churn out in 400-metre reps. That upper gear has been missing for months, come to think of it ... maybe a year. Or maybe more?

I'll tell you what else disturbs me. These shorts. The same company I've been getting my running clobber from for the last decade has definitely started making them tighter at the waist. Yikes! When I look down, for the first time in my running life, despite being careful with cake and biscuits, I've actually got a muffin top. As I (breathlessly) jog past some pensioners, I scream, 'I don't normally look like this – they've changed the sizes!' In my head.

Okay, full confession time: when I say I'm in my prime, that might be a little bit of fairy dust. Though I have the haircut of a seventeen-year-old who's just lost a drunken fight with a lawnmower, technically I'm fifty. But today is the first day in my life that I've categorically felt ...

Old.

There. I said it.

Ouch.

A few weeks later I run a local, 12-kilometre trail race called Over The Hills and place fourteenth in 48:30. Second V40 or OG (old git). Not bad, I guess. But I've won that race. Twice. And here's the glaringly significant thing: I used to run it three minutes faster. Albeit that was five years ago.

My age-category placing used to be something I'd look down my nose at, like a bonus Easter egg left over from the main hunt. First V40, too? Nice. But I didn't really care. Now it's all I care about.

I felt uncomfortably grown-up when I found myself in a nightclub on my fortieth birthday and all the music sounded too loud and samey. I also felt like an imposter of an adult when my eldest child graduated from primary to secondary school. When you're twelve years into being a parent, you can't really claim to be a new one any more. You're no longer an accidental grown-up just muddling through, still believing you're twenty-seven in spirit, still at Glastonbury festival, the numbers beside your age on forms just a silly admin error. And let's not get started on why my unfaithful follicles have decided it's much more fun to grow hair out of my nose, shoulders and ears than on my actual head. I'll never forgive that cruel mutiny.

I guess this is what ageing feels like. I don't like it one bit, but I guess I need to admit that it really is happening. I'm ageing. There's no hiding from the depressing truth that I'm officially past my best. Over The Hills has shown me, with a crushing irony, that I am now over the hill. It's a big moment, realising. Till then, life had felt like it was on an upward trajectory, or at least a flat line, perhaps. Now I'm staring at a downward slope, the void clawing at me. Getting older sucks already. And I've only just got started.

There's some really good news coming, I promise. But in some ways, running, more than most sports, makes ageing a harrowing experience. We have such measurable, standardised performance, at parkrun, at a marathon or even just going out and running a mile on a flat road as fast as we ruddy well can. Our decline is shoved in our face on every run. And while one of the tenets of run coaching is to not read too much into one session, perhaps we do it twice or over a period of those increasingly precious weeks and months. And we can see quite easily and starkly the athletic and human decline. Those exact same data points, calculated by that clever gadget on our wrist, that gave us such motivational joy in those glorious early days of being a runner, now savagely mock our feeble efforts. 'Ha, is that all you've got? Face it. You're slow(er) and old(er).'

Of course, running is about so much more than numbers, but my watch has gone from something I turn to for reassurance of my prowess, confirmation of my potency, to something, frankly, I don't want to look at. I don't need a small piece of technology telling me I'm past my best-before date. Plus, there are probably some GPS blackspots around here anyway.

My body tells me, too. With niggles in my foot and my Achilles tendon that never quite go away. Tightness in my calf that is apathetic towards foam rolling. A weird discomfort in my shoulder that's been there for two years (probably something to do with working too many hours at a laptop – we'll get on to that – the act of writing this book didn't help). Three-minute hills just feel harder. Fast runs feel like the same effort as ever, but my watch says they're less fast. Easy runs sometimes don't feel easy. I really need my sleep now. I feel tired. I didn't use to be so tired. Or wrinkly.

It's not just athletic performance. Society, too, doesn't need us like it did. *Last of the Summer Wine, Dad's Army* – they don't seem funny now. Nor those HILARIOUS birthday cards. Indeed, the UK's advertising standards watchdog recently criticised the use of negative and even offensive portrayals of older people in commercials, stereotyping them as lonely, intolerant and grumpy. Bah!

'Old: it's a withering label, loaded with far more meaning and judgement than the bald [pun unintended] fact you were born long ago,' writes Richard Askwith in the excellent *The Race Against Time*. 'Among much else, it suggests irrelevance, as if the part of your life that mattered had already been lived. Your story is in the past, not the future.'

In truth, my body has been good to me. While I've never had the height, hair or muscles I would have liked, I've run up and down mountains, bimbled for hundreds of miles at a time, and yet haven't had any major physical or health setbacks (though chicken pox was rough). While my body isn't letting me down in a chronic way yet, there is an undeniable decline. It's clear that I'm just not as powerful, fast or durable as I was. I'm a little bit slower, less robust, and a bit more flabby and lumpy in the wrong places. My body is just not as, well, *good* as it once was. I don't like it. But I guess it's time to face up to it and see what can be done to lessen the fade.

Technically, I've been a veteran or masters athlete for almost a decade. Nothing changed at first. Having rediscovered the deep and addictive joy of running aged thirty-six and as a new parent, I'm something of a late starter. Those initial few years were glorious, full of PBs and the joy of accomplishing ouchy but deeply satisfying new distances.

I became one of those annoying running evangelists, thinking everyone should just go for a run and they'd find true enlightenment and running would save the world. After a first marathon, I realised people did the same thing on trails and often went much, much further, and I got carried away.

It wasn't long before I was running 100-mile mountain races such as UTMB Mont-Blanc, the 200-plus-mile Dragon's Back Race, the 268-mile Winter Spine Race. I became competitive, setting records/Fastest Known Times on National Trails and fell-running rounds, and was once even selected for the GB trail running team, aged forty (I wrote a separate book about all that).

My best objective performance, fifth place at UTMB, the Super Bowl of ultra-trail running, was at the age of forty-two. For my other most notable performance, breaking the record for the Pennine Way, I was forty-four. It was after winning the 2023 Winter Spine Race three years later that I was first officially called a 'veteran' in a write-up, which made me wince. As we'll see, both anecdotally and scientifically, seniority matters less the longer the race and is actually an advantage.

However, in the 2024 Winter Spine Race, I had my wrinkly butt well and truly kicked by Jack Scott, an athlete literally young enough to be my son. He's a good friend and we've met for training runs through the years, but the transfer of power is very much in evidence on those now too. I'm not getting any younger. (I've always hated that phrase. No one is.)

I've thought about those contrasting two years a lot. They felt like they may have represented my peak and the beginning of the end for me as an elite athlete (thankfully, that's turned out to be poppycock). The thing is, with the caveat that the Spine Race is far from a typical running event, it was the 2022 race I should have seen as more noteworthy.

I was also in that year's event and I was in first place after halfway. But my relative inexperience in leading races caused me to misjudge my effort and push unnecessarily hard; a dull ache became a sharp pain and I dropped out of the race, fearing for the long-term implications. So too did the younger runner behind me. This allowed Irishman Eoin Keith to move into pole position and take the win, aged fifty-three, having previously been back in fifteenth place.

When asked about his tactics, Eoin said, 'to run my own race. It was my most comfortable and balanced Spine Race. I don't have gear 5 any more, but I've always said if you run your own race and optimise your own performance, your best performance will come out.'

A masterful lesson in midlife running for us all. Also, in two out of those three years at the Winter Spine Race, the male winner was in their late forties or early fifties. And while I write this, the extraordinary Anna Troup, aged fifty-five, has just won the Summer Spine Race overall, after three years of injury (more from her on page 134; and more from Eoin on page 91). I hope this book shows runners that in some ways what Anna did shouldn't be that extraordinary. We can all be ageless aces. There are some incredibly inspiring runners and performances in this book, giving us all hope.

However, there will be people reading this with growing annoyance, thinking, *fifty isn't old, matey; just you wait till [insert age here] – you're in for a shock*. And indeed at the 2025 National Running Show, Angela White, aka The Running Granny, the oldest woman to run 875 miles from John o'Groats to Land's End, rightly reprimanded me for calling myself old. 'You're not old,' she said. 'You're just older.' Which feels like an important difference.

This book came about because I wanted to find out what was happening to me as a runner and as a person as I aged. I thought that there must be thousands of runners going through the same thing. I wanted to understand the physiological changes: what exactly is happening to me? But I also wanted to see if any could be slowed, paused or even reversed – and, to my great joy, many can. I found some useful books on the subject, but none that spoke directly to me as a midlife runner.

I really wanted to know how fast my athletic and health decline is forecast to be. What exactly are the physiological changes as we age and how do they affect my athleticism? Which aspects of running fitness might go quickest and which might last longest? Which could be worked on to maintain them? Should I train differently? Do injury-avoidance strategies need to change? Do I need to start pumping iron (yuk), lifting actual barbells instead of half-heartedly swinging a kettlebell about a bit? How about my diet and sleep? Does my mindset matter at all? But as well as all the potential downsides and new things I might need to be doing, are there any advantages to being a mature athlete? Spoiler alert: heck yeah!

The more I read about ageing, the more words like 'longevity' kept popping up, and the links between running and health. I couldn't help but think and worry about my lifespan and, more importantly, my healthspan. If I can carry on running through middle age and beyond, how concerned should I be about the Four Horsemen of the Apocalypse: cardiovascular disease, diabetes, dementia and cancer? More importantly, is it optimally healthy to continue with my eleven-cups-a-day tea addiction?

In researching this book, I was horrified to discover just how comprehensive ageing is and all the things I'm about to die from. Paradoxically, though, I've been thrilled to find just how much we can stick a middle finger up at time and rage against age. These discoveries are highly motivating. I've learned many things – some alarming, some reassuring, some surprising, some outlandish. But above all, I learned we definitely can claw back some significant control over how we age – as athletes and as people. But most of us need to change some things up. Us old(er) dogs need to learn some new tricks.

I'm going to share how to train to be a kick-ass masters runner, a midlife maestro, an ageless ace. This has huge knock-on health benefits, which should greatly interest most midlife people; with parents well into their seventies, it's doubly interesting.

It may sound dramatic, but some of the information in here could save lives and make those final decades much more enjoyable. We can indeed extend our healthspans. And it doesn't involve taking seventy-two daily supplements, ice barrel submersions or licking toads.

We're at a new frontier of science and practice for both health and performance. The generation before us didn't have the knowledge we have now or the socialised motivations to rage against the dying of the light. Our parents weren't out running 100-milers, sportives and Ironmans into their forties, fifties, sixties and beyond, because they were told it would wreck their knees or kill them. We are. In running and other sports, we've seen extraordinary performances from veteran athletes, which is kicking the science along. Ageing is inevitable. *How we age* isn't.

Other books on the topic are largely written by men for men. As I can only change one of those equations on my own, I've brought in world-renowned sports dietitian, author and kick-ass ultrarunner Renee

McGregor, fifty, to explain how ageing affects female runners, especially around the ironically named menopause. I'm also grateful to record-breaking lifter, strength and conditioning coach, and sub-three-hour-marathoner Pete Stables for sharing his expertise, enthusiasm and wit. I can only apologise to trans people as there just doesn't seem to be any good research on sport and ageing on this demographic yet.

This feels like as good a moment as any to discuss words, their power and what we should we call ourselves. 'Masters athlete', the US version, sounds infinitely better to me than the UK version, 'veteran', which is basically another disparaging word for 'old'. It also implies a lot has happened, when I much prefer a focus on all the things we can do now and all the adventures ahead of us. So the word 'veteran' is banned from this book and I've limited use of the word 'old', too. Language has power, it makes a difference. We may be a little bit *older* than some, but not necessarily *old.* We're in our middle age or midlife – our prime, quite frankly. 'Mature' has a whiff of advantage to it too, of reaching a kind of potential or fullness. And I know I'm not alone in still wanting to attempt big things, try new types of running, have fresh adventures. There are some incredible, inspiring, ageless aces interviewed in this book who are doing just that. Plus, as they discuss, age – or perhaps more accurately, *experience* – is a huge advantage.

While we may not be at our fastest, I like to think we're in our very best years, our optimal time. And we value them more because we know how precious they are. We're not running out of time. We're using our time to run. And to properly live.

I've accepted that I used to be faster, but that hasn't affected the simple fact that I still just ruddy love running. For freedom, for adventure, for health, for time with friends old and new, and purely for the sake of the gloriously simple act of running. I love it for the smelly clothes and wet feet, for bramble scratches and grazed knees, for mud up my calves and sweat on my lips. Though I've reluctantly admitted my athletic potential has been realised, I like to think I'm still in it and will do all I can to stay in it. I'm determined to maximise my running till I have to be scraped up off the tarmac or trail by people in white coats.

I'm going to run forever.

PART ONE: THE BAD

'As you get older, three things happen. The first is your memory goes, and I can't remember the other two.'

SIR NORMAN WISDOM

This section is on reflection a bit depressing. If you'd rather not know all the things about to go wrong with you, feel free to jump to *Part Two: The Good*, on page 17, which is much more cheery. But if you insist on knowing, let's look into what happens to us, as runners and as people, as we age. First, let's look at when and why humans age. 'At some point, your body will decide to grow senescent [your cells start dying] and then to die,' sums up Bill Bryson, father-in-law incidentally to an elite ultrarunner, in *The Body: A Guide for Occupants*. Thanks, Bill.

When is that point? Some early ageing starts in our twenties, related to metabolism, but it's barely detectable. Physiologically, we *Homo sapiens* are past our peak at the blissfully naive age of thirty. Youth, eh? Wasted on the young. In the general population, forty-four and sixty may be significant ageing cliffs, according to a 2024 Stanford study of thousands of different molecules and microbiomes in 108 people aged 25–75 – so two 'massive biomolecular shifts', rather than a gradual phasing out.[1] But research on runners suggests a different pattern and we'll get on to what actually happens to us. But first, why does ageing happen?

Ageing is best understood as a trade-off between cell maintenance and reproduction, says Nobel Prize-winning molecular biologist Venki Ramakrishnan, author of *Why We Die: The New Science of Ageing and the Quest for Immortality*. Evolution selects for growing fast and maturing quickly, so we can get on with reproducing and passing along genes. Initially, our bodies use their resources for growth, health and survival. At sexual maturity, the priority switches to reproducing. After sexual maturity, look out. We've served our purpose. The force of natural selection weakens and the ageing process begins, leading ultimately to death.

The salmon, for example, is able to make the long arduous journey swimming upstream to spawn, then promptly dies afterwards. All its cells work to give it the best chance of getting to the spawning ground and making the most of the opportunity. But the chances of it swimming back downstream, surviving another year at sea, making the same return trip and successfully spawning again are slim and natural selection doesn't favour them. Indeed, most animals die soon after they lose the ability to reproduce. Homo sapiens, thankfully, do not. In fact, women spend around a third of their lives in a postmenopausal state and we're among very few species – joining sheep, chimps and two types of whale – who continue past that key phase.

For most mammals, the larger the animal, the longer the lifespan. Scientist Steven Austad studies the relationship between size and longevity in animals. He invented the longevity quotient, which shows that humans actually live five times longer than expected, only outperformed by eighteen species of bat and the naked mole-rat (technically neither mole nor rat). The naked mole-rat is studied a lot, because it seems to be cancer-resistant and demonstrates negligible senescence. Its mortality does not increase with age. We all want to be more naked mole-rat.

The hydra is another outlier. This small aquatic animal regenerates tissue continuously and doesn't seem to age at all; while one jellyfish species is often labelled immortal because when faced with injury or stress, it metamorphoses into an earlier version and lives its life all over again.

Lifespans of organisms range from a few hours for some unlucky insects to hundreds of years for some whales, giant tortoises (both around 200) and Greenland sharks (400), to 5,000 years for bristlecone pine trees.

So some biologists live in hope that ageing and death for us aren't inevitable. But so far, it has always happened.

Age-old debate

From around the age of thirty, we're in a race against time. But it used to be much worse. For most of human history, life expectancy – the average years a person is likely to live for at their birth – was just thirty, by which age we were usually grandparents and had largely served our evolutionary purpose. We could still be semi-helpful for gathering berries, free babysitting and telling dad/grandad jokes. But we could also be an extra mouth to feed when food was scarce.

Why do we live for so much longer after sexual maturity nowadays? The grandmother hypothesis suggests it's important for older relatives to stay alive because reproduction is a risky business. A grandmother can ensure the survival of some of her own genes by investing in her grandchildren, so longer life could bring an advantage from a natural selection point of view. The good news for women is that they've always outlived men and are ten times more likely to reach 110. That said, women have to contend with myriad complications from the menopause, typically starting from the age of forty-five but it can be much earlier (renowned sports dietitian Renee McGregor writes about mastering menopause on page 48).

A hundred years ago, we could expect to live into our forties in the UK, and even in 1950 it was into our sixties. Improvements in public health, primarily sanitation and sterilisation of water and food, rather than groundbreaking advancements in medicine, have had the biggest impact, dramatically reducing infant mortality rates – though vaccines, antibiotics, blood transfusions and, surprisingly, fertilisers have played significant roles, too. Today, life expectancy is 81, though one in six babies born now can expect to live to 100. Compared to our ancestors, we've essentially been given a second life. So perhaps we shouldn't be too gloomy and ungrateful about sliding further away from that parkrun PB.

The big question that causes big squabbles amongst biologists is whether there's a theoretical maximum lifespan for humans, or – if we dodge the worst diseases, drunk drivers and lightning – can we just carry on indefinitely? Because of some of the miraculous lifespans of other species, some biologists do not think ageing is inevitable and there's theoretically no evidence for a limit on human lifespan. Some argue the first human to live to 150 is already alive. Some argue that's all codswallop. But the idea is enough to trigger a few tech millionaires to push for immortality (more on page 169).

Tellingly, perhaps, while life expectancy has doubled in a short space of time, maximum human lifespan – the oldest age reached – hasn't grown. The oldest recorded human, Italy's Jeanne Louise Calment, endured to see her 122nd birthday. She was a smoker and ate lots of chocolate. But she also had only one child, never had a job as such or financial worries for most of her life and was active every day, enjoying bike rides. (Ahem, though there are rumours her daughter may have assumed her identity at some point.)

We used to die younger and faster, mostly from infection or trauma. Now we die older and slower, usually from lifestyle diseases. **Two thirds of the world's population die from age-related causes, the Four Horsemen of the Apocalypse**: the ticking time bombs of cardiovascular disease, neurodegenerative disease, diabetes and cancer. Though we live on average twice as long as we did 150 years ago, we spend a much greater percentage of our lives in decline, functioning at less than 50% of our capacity. In the US, **80% of adults will have a chronic health condition by the time they're sixty-five – the early signs of which can be present in our twenties.** In the UK, the average male will spend sixteen years in poor health, the average female twenty years, according to a recent study.[2]

Cellular data

Though it makes good sense evolutionarily, on a biological level, scientists aren't exactly sure why we age. There are lots of ideas – some 300, in fact – and they fall into three main theories: cellular waste accumulation theories (your cells fill up with toxic waste by-products), genetic mutation theories (your genes malfunction and, um, terminate you) and, the one that sounds more realistic to runners, wear-and-tear theories (your body simply wears out). What scientists do feel certain of is that this happens inside us, in our cells.

Over the course of our lives, our genes collect mutations. Some are completely random, others the result of our diets or external factors such as UV light. Very few are useful, most do nothing, but some are harmful. Before sexual maturity, any gene mutation that decreases an organism's likelihood to reproduce is strongly selected against. But once an organism reaches sexual maturity, there's little benefit in continuing the effort required to stay healthy and senescence, or cellular ageing, starts.

Before sexual maturity, stem cells divide to repair and replace parts of our body, such as those gene mutations. But when senescence hits, those same cells turn on us and mutiny. More recently termed 'zombie cells', they're no longer capable of dividing and can negatively impact the cells around them, weakening our tissues, organs and immune system. BRCA gene mutations are a classic example. They are linked to higher fertility in women, but also significantly increase the risk of breast and ovarian cancers. Stem cells protect us against cancer by preventing cells with DNA damage from multiplying, but senescent cells can accumulate in tissues, causing damage and inflammation, precursors to age-related illnesses. Stem cell repair works really well for a time, but deteriorates with age and eventually the cells down tools. (In more positive news, in March 2025 scientists from Dundee University claimed to have discovered a way to identify and eliminate zombie cells.[3])

Telomeres, stretches of specialised DNA at the end of each chromosome, shorten with each cell division, working as a type of tallying device. Eventually, they reach a predetermined length – which varies from one cell type to another – and the cells become inactive or die. The length of our telomeres (not that we can see them) is a key internal sign of our biological ageing. We'll learn more about this later.

What does ageing look like? In biological-speak, the twelve hallmarks of ageing, according to a 2023 study, are:

- cellular senescence
- stem cell exhaustion
- mitochondrial dysfunction
- telomere attrition
- chronic inflammation

- genomic instability
- epigenetic alterations
- loss of proteostasis
- disabled macroautophagy
- deregulated nutrient-sensing
- altered intercellular communication
- dysbiosis.[4]

Some of that may not mean much (to me included, until recently), but you'll probably agree that it doesn't sound particularly promising. The news that ageing is bobbins won't be entirely unexpected, but the full picture could be worse than we imagined. It affects *everything*. There is some good news coming for us runners. But to understand all of that, we first need to understand what's happening to us as runners.

The race against time

Most athletes towards the end of their forties will have probably felt they're just not as fast as they once were. One of the earliest and most upsetting physiological declines is deteriorating lung function as the air sacs that make up our lungs lose their elasticity. The headline is that **our VO2 max,** the maximum oxygen uptake we can manage during physical exertion, **declines by around 7–10% per decade, from as early as thirty**. So a seventy-year-old has lost about 25% of their aerobic horsepower compared to their forty-year-old self. That feels huge. And demoralising. As we'll see, though, the decline can be less for us runners.

In news that may sound like it's good for us joggers but bad for our sedentary friends, nothing dictates our lifespan and healthspan (the quality of our life, not just its length) like our VO2 max does. Essentially, several studies have shown that the fittest people have the lowest mortality rates, and by a surprising margin. Someone in the bottom quartile of VO2 max for their age group is four times more likely to die than an elite-level runner. Even improving VO2 max from the bottom 25% into the 25th–50th percentile cuts the risk of death by half. Poor cardiorespiratory fitness carries a greater relative risk than smoking.

Depressingly, our heart is going to shrink and stiffen. Our cardiac capacity or maximal heart rate – the highest rate we can reach, when running fast – drops off. There is a steady fall in the number of receptors in our heart muscle listening to the nervous system's signals and telling it how fast to beat. As the heart becomes increasingly deaf to these messages, its maximum rate drops. There also appears to be a decline in the heart's intrinsic ability to beat quickly, but it's actually that the heart can't relax – or, in running speak, 'recover' – as quickly as it used to. Most of us can hit 200 beats per minute (bpm) on short intervals in early adulthood, but **from around thirty the heart's peak capacity to pump blood declines by 1 bpm per year or 5–10% per decade**. The heart's vitality doesn't decline as steeply as lung function, but as less oxygen is delivered to the bloodstream and muscles, there's a corresponding decline in our running performance. As overall blood volume is reduced, our organs get less blood, too. We also have less muscle (more anon), fewer mitochondria (the powerhouses of our muscles), perhaps fewer capillaries, and our arteries may become clogged and/or inelastic.

In further bad but not hugely unexpected news, our lactate threshold also decreases, reducing the intensity we can sustain or our speed endurance. These physiological processes – heart, blood, lungs, lactate threshold – are all linked to one another, are all key to athletic performance and are all on the wane. In summary, as we age, we runners simply can't go as fast as we used to. It's both a physical and an existential crisis. And it's really frustrating.

Weakly mileage

Looking at the elite pen at the start of the London Marathon, a non-runner would be forgiven for thinking that muscles and strength weren't high on a runner's priority list. And they'd probably be right (Kenyan runners don't tend to do strength work). But reaching masters status as a runner has big implications for our muscles. Or lack thereof. Around 20% of adults will experience sarcopenia, age-related skeletal muscle atrophy or muscle wastage. 'Like a snowman in a thaw,' writes Richard Askwith in *The Race Against Time*.

Even if we dodge sarcopenia, we will lose individual muscle fibres and – unlike hair, nails and white blood cells – we can't grow new ones. They atrophy and die. **Muscles can start waving their little white flags as early as twenty-five.** We decline more definitely from around forty and it's much clearer after fifty, where men lose 1–2% of muscle mass each year and 3% each year after sixty. By the age of eighty a man can have said goodbye to a whopping 50% of the muscle mass he had at twenty-five. That's huge – or rather, we won't be. Women lose less muscle mass, around 3–5% per decade from the age of thirty (more anon).

Mass, however, is the least important metric here. **We lose muscle *strength* two to three times faster** than we lose mass. **And we lose muscle *power*** – best understood as the speed at which force is produced – earlier and **two to three times faster than we lose strength**. It drops by 2–4% per year.

This muscle wastage places an abnormal load on tendons and ligaments, which can lead to injury. Crucially, we tend to lose fast-twitch muscle fibres more quickly than slow-twitch fibres, leaving us with weaker and less explosive muscles overall. Simply staying fit isn't enough to keep those fast-twitch fibres firing. Power, or the ability to deliver force quickly, is the number-one factor that separates young athletes from older ones, writes Jeff Bercovici in *Play On: The New Science of Elite Performance at Any Age*.

Even if we maintain the same muscle mass, **our muscles fatigue more quickly as we age. Our body becomes less efficient at delivering nutrition to muscles** (known as protein synthesis), making it harder to rebuild them through exercise (known as anabolic resistance). The body has to work harder to convert protein into muscle fibres, so a sedentary sixty-year-old will have to do twice the resistance training of a sedentary twenty-year-old to get the same result. DOMS (delayed-onset muscle soreness) can last longer. At some point **our muscles actually start to work against us.** 'Co-activation of the antagonist muscle' means that when we try a bicep curl, the tricep is firing too, resisting the movement. Balance and coordination are also affected.

It's not just athletics and aesthetics. Health-wise, **muscles protect us from disease**. Muscle is the predominant sink for glucose uptake, so the more skeletal muscle we have, the more easily we can maintain low blood sugar, putting off the Four Horsemen and other unwanted health outcomes. In late midlife, the real problem is the loss of the ability to move well, respond quickly to say a trip or stumble and even remain independent. Everyday lifestyle things such as carrying food shopping, lifting a grandchild or getting up from a chair unaided become difficult or no longer possible. Falls become more likely and can have very serious implications.

One in three people aged sixty-five or older fall each year and **falling is the second leading cause of unintentional injury deaths worldwide,** after road traffic accidents. Falls are responsible for over 38 million DALYs (disability-adjusted life years) and result in more years lived with disability than transport injury, drowning, burns and poisoning combined. Fewer than 50% of patients who suffer hip fractures in older age return to full pre-fall function, and 30% of hip fracture patients die within the first year of their injury.

Even if a fall is less directly impactful health-wise, people lose confidence, become less active and are less likely to do things they enjoy doing, negatively impacting mental health. Poor balance at fifty is a strong indicator of our risk of falls at seventy, found a 2022 study. **Adults aged 51–75 who couldn't stand on one leg for ten seconds had nearly twice the risk of dying over the next seven years.**[5] Though the reasons for falls are multi-factorial and eyesight is certainly up there, lack of strength, balance and bone health (and vitamin D deficiency) are key. That spectre is hopefully a while further down the line for most of us, but it feels like something we should warn our parents about now.

The bones of it

Talking of bone health, **up to 50% of women and 25% of men aged fifty-plus will break a bone.** The calcium-rich white things we rely on as part of our skeleton get weaker as the years tick by, with serious ramifications. We become increasingly susceptible to osteoporosis, which weakens our bones, making them more likely to fracture and break. When hormones plummet around menopause, bone strength declines by 10–20% and fractures rocket up from the late forties onwards. For women, the incidence of broken bones is greater than that of heart attack, stroke and breast cancer combined. Later, that can be the beginning of the end.

Osteoporosis is an imbalance between how much of our bones is being renewed and how much is being absorbed by the rest of the body. Our bones are continuously transferring minerals into our blood to facilitate key bodily processes, a natural cycle of regeneration. But if there's not enough calcium doing the rounds, the body will simply steal more of it from our bones to fill the gap, leaving them weaker. Broken bones take longer to knit back together the older we get and **people with poor bone health are also more likely to have dementia.**[6] Runners with a lower BMI or who've had REDs (relative energy deficiency in sport), an eating disorder or disordered eating are more at risk of poor bone health.

We reach peak bone mineral density (BMD) at about thirty, depending on diet and lifestyle, when women have about 125 grams of skeletal calcium, men 150 grams. The decline in BMD for men is fairly constant, but for women the decline steepens around menopause and especially at the age of fifty, then levels off around sixty. Sweating and dehydration also negatively affect our bone mineral density, as does our diet if there's not enough calcium or vitamin D going in (more on page 139).

We can easily take our skeleton for granted. It's the strong, silent type, just an overpowered coat hanger for our skin and muscles. But our skeleton isn't just structural, it's our body's 'master communicator', says Dr Vonda Wright, an orthopaedic surgeon and author of *Unbreakable: A Woman's Guide to Ageing with Power*. Our bones release proteins and talk to our brain via hormones such as osteocalcin. Stimulating bones helps build neurons, metabolise glucose and make testosterone.

Hormonally not yours

We get whacked another time by the giant ageing mallet. The endocrine system plays a vital role in keeping us in physiological equilibrium or homeostasis. The endocrine system uses chemical messaging to signal when some biochemical rebalancing is required. For example, in a stressful situation, if a threat is perceived – the obvious example being a sixteen-year-old chasing us down at parkrun – the adrenal glands signal that adrenaline is required and ask the heart rate and blood pressure to work harder and speed us to the finish faster. Hormones tell us when to eat and sleep, create desire to have sex, make us feel happy or sad, even communicate when to grow. They're really important. But most hormone levels decline as we age, in particular those which help us adapt to training.

Both men and women have the sex hormone oestrogen, but it's more prevalent and powerful in women, whereas men have significantly more testosterone. Oestrogen drops off a cliff during a menopausal state and is more complex and nuanced than testosterone decline in men, which is also more linear. For women this means:

- bone mineral density decline
- loss of anti-inflammatory qualities which aid the immune system
- loss of heart protection, especially during high-level endurance activity
- interrupted and loss of quality sleep
- more visceral and belly fat.

Men in turn lose testosterone, with big implications for athletic performance and health. Both sexes have testosterone and it declines (I don't know about you, but I'm getting fed up of that word) by about 1% per year in men from the age of thirty. By their seventies and eighties, men have only about half the levels they had in their twenties. Diminishing testosterone in men leads to:

- osteopenia and osteoporosis – loss of bone strength
- sarcopenia – age-related muscle loss
- increased lipid stores – i.e. more body fat
- lower libido – declining sex drive
- declining cognitive function – alertness and sharpness both drop.

Levels of testosterone are also the key difference between the sexes, helping to make men stronger and faster (and perhaps more ego-driven and worse at pacing marathons). It's also one of the popular ways to dope, so ageing is effectively the opposite of doping.

A weighting game

Many symptoms of ageing are linked to declining testosterone levels. For example, the less testosterone you have, the harder it is to maintain and build skeletal muscle. That muscle burns a lot of calories. As you lose it, your metabolism slows, meaning those calories are more likely to turn into fat on your waist. Fat secretes oestrogen and proteins that promote chronic inflammation and insulin resistance. 'Ageing makes us fat, and then fat makes us age,' writes Bill Gifford in *Spring Chicken*.

As well as the extra expense of new running shorts in a bigger size and the increasingly displeasing morning appearance in a full-length mirror, excess weight erodes our efforts to maintain optimal VO_2 max and primary muscles have to work harder just to maintain the same pace, needing more oxygen to do so. Increased lipoprotein lipase (LPL) fat could also be reducing insulin sensitivity. Testosterone used to help keep stores at bay, but we have less of it now. Added weight brings down our VO_2 max too, so we get slower. It's a depressing spiral.

The human growth hormone (HGH) is the third crucial hormone for athleticism and health. It's so influential in our bodies that searching for illicit supplements of it is the number-one target for the World Anti-Doping Agency. HGH is released as we sleep (more about sleep on page 124), signalling growth receptor cells all around the body to reproduce and grow, making us bigger, stronger and physically more capable. HGH peaks during puberty and declines by 1–2% per year after the age of thirty. HGH decline is related to:

- decrease in lean muscle bulk
- increase in both body lipids (fats) and visceral fats
- reduction in aerobic capacity (VO_2 max)
- decrease in bone mineral formation
- decrease in natural EPO production in the kidneys
- neural decline – possibly affecting cognition and alertness
- deterioration of the immune system.

Melatonin and insulin are crucial hormones that also deplete as we age and impact our metabolism. Melatonin is related to our sleep and our circadian rhythms. It's secreted from the pineal gland, which is large in children, but shrinks post-puberty and becomes further compromised as we get older. Essentially, quality sleep is harder to come by in later years.

Insulin, meanwhile, decreases the glucose levels in our blood, but after fifty our body becomes less efficient at metabolising it, meaning greater sensitivity to sugar, higher levels of glucose and increased risk of diabetes. Indeed, the typical age of a type 2 diabetes diagnosis is between forty-five and sixty-four, with men at higher risk, black and southern-Asian men even more so.

Achy breaky parts

Notice how recovery feels slower in your groaning hips and ankles? Ageing also changes the biology, healing capacity and biomechanical function of tendons and ligaments, both somewhat important to runners, with implications for our joints, too. Connective tissue loses its elasticity and muscles get tight, a one–two punch that can cause injury and force a shortened stride, slowing us down and reducing our running economy.

Most runners will have had some sort of tendon issue at some point, with Achilles tendonitis being a popular and tenacious niggle (I can attest to that). Tendons join muscle to bones, while ligaments join bone to bone. Both are fibrous connective tissue that aids joint motion and stability. Tendons and ligaments make joints work and we know range of motion also reduces with age. Think of them losing elasticity, becoming more fragile and a little more disorganised, and the chances of running injury increasing as a result.

Whether it's tendons and fascia, tighter muscles, and/or a bit of something else, we know that **reduced range of motion, flexibility, mobility, balance, proprioception and overall recovery rate are all things that affect the more mature athlete.**

All injuries, from bruises to tendon strains, take longer to heal, which is thought to be something to do with the deteriorating function of the specialised stem cells that carry out repairs and the decreasing production of growth hormones. This also means slower recovery and adaptations from more challenging training.

Nerve function also deteriorates. The pace at which nerve signals travel around the body to create reaction times declines gradually from the age of twenty-four. As motor neurons die, motor units become less efficient, meaning progressive loss of balance and greater risk of injury, both when running and when not running.

As if all of that wasn't enough for the mature runner to contend with, **our immune system becomes less efficient, making colds and worse things more likely**, meaning more interruptions to training. This can speed our decline up just that little bit more.

Wait, there's more. As we get into our latter decades, we'll find our bladders have become less elastic, hence why we find ourselves increasingly pausing our watches on long runs. Skin also loses elasticity, getting more leathery and drier (so it wasn't just another dehydrated run). Blood vessels are less robust, breaking more easily and causing more bruises. We'll get into fat in more detail, but at the latter end of things, the fat close to skin actually thins, making it harder for elderly folk to stay warm. And we technically shrink, up to two inches by the age of eighty, due to compressed spinal discs.

We also experience changes in our brain (cognitive decline and memory loss), kidneys, hearing, eyesight, hair (come back, you gits!) and libido. Osteoarthritis, a painful inflammation of the bones and joints, becomes more common as the cartilage that acts as a shock absorber wears down and the cells that help it grow get worse at their job. I don't know about you, but at the moment it feels like ageing is a highly overrated idea.

The midlife crisis

Not all changes are physical. Have you had your midlife crisis yet? Considering a short trip to Turkey, buying a Tesla or dabbling in CrossFit are all sure signs. The midlife crisis is a relatively new construct – unsurprising perhaps when we only used to live to thirty.

Aristotle believed middle age to be the prime of our life, having reached peak competence and mastery. In the 1960s the idea that midlife was the period from forty to sixty where we pondered our mortality became prevalent, probably stemming from Canadian psychoanalyst Elliott Jaques.

A 2008 paper titled 'Is well-being U-shaped over the life cycle?' suggested that happiness is high in youth, dips significantly in the mid- to late forties, and then ends up high again in older age.

A midlife crisis feels like a real thing. It could well be the rise of FOMO coupled with the panicky idea that we don't have much time left to get on with all these possibilities, suggests Gwendolyn Bounds in *Not Too Late: The Power of Pushing Limits at Any Age*. Essentially, it can feel like there's so much to do and so little time, which makes us anxious. Having so many options is actually making us unhappy. This 'crisis' throws some people into running, and if that's you, welcome. You made a great choice.

In summary

For the runner, if we do nothing to counteract age decline, we get weaker, slower and less powerful. Our bodies whinge, hurt and break more easily. Recovery from workouts (intervals and other high-intensity running), races and injury is just slower. And those injuries are more likely. Interruptions from training accelerate the decline. As a consequence, motivation can take a hit. Concurrently, work and family 'get in the way'. It all doom-spirals together and suddenly we're not just old but prematurely old, speeding towards the race finish line we don't want to reach.

In a summary we all don't want to read, the big initial changes faced by both sexes as we age are decreased cardiac output, stoke volume and maximal heart rate; decreased aerobic (VO_2) output; diminishment of the sport-critical sex hormones oestrogen in women and testosterone in men; reduced mitochondrial efficiency (energy production) and arterial stiffness. Muscles waste away from as young as thirty and we could get 8% weaker per decade. This accelerates around sixty (which also means less glycogen storage among other bad things), limiting performance and recovery. Our fast-twitch fibres go first; our bones also get weaker; our tendons, ligaments and joints are all less happy; our balance, coordination and flexibility all decline; our metabolism becomes less effective and we get fatter; and our sleep gets worse.

Outside of running, our hearing and eyesight diminish. We get saggier and wrinklier, with less hair in the places society deems attractive and more in the places it doesn't. Importantly and frustratingly, these factors all feed off each other in the ultimate doom spiral, accelerating our ageing and leading to further deterioration for both athletic and general health, making us more susceptible to other, much more serious, issues.

In almost every way you think about it, getting older is rubbish physiologically. However, as well as celebrating what all those extra years on Earth gift us and all the accrued wisdom and photos, we do have a surprising level of control over many of these unwanted facets of ageing. We can slow, pause and even reverse them. Ageing is inevitable. *How* we age is a choice.

PART TWO: THE GOOD

'Do not go gentle into that good night,
Old age should burn and rave at close of day,
Rage, rage against the dying of the light.'

DYLAN THOMAS

So, we've established beyond all reasonable doubt that getting older, from a biological perspective, is really rubbish. But here is some good news. A lot of it.

Biological ageing

Our chronological age and our biological age are two very different things. Our chronological age is simply how many years we've been on Earth. Our biological age, however, is a much more malleable and exciting concept.

The unstoppable march of time doesn't intrude on us all equally. We age at different rates and in different ways. Some of that is genetic, but probably less than you might think (more anon). One of the key factors is environmental – for example, smoking, alcohol, sleep, diet, stress, social isolation and overexposure to the sun are all linked to accelerated biological ageing. The same is true of repeated exposure to the heatwaves which are now more common due to the climate crisis, reported a 2025 study, with a negative health impact broadly comparable with the damage caused by smoking, alcohol or a poor diet.[1]

We know that the kidneys, liver, metabolism and immune system age at different rates in different people. When tissue is removed from both breast and brain cancer patients, it tends to have a biological age older than its owners' chronological age, says Dr Morgan Levine, Head of Aging at Yale University's Living Systems Lab and author of *True Age*. 'Biological age – not chronological age – is what underlies the changes we see in the mirror,' she says. 'The biological changes we feel as we rise out of bed each morning. The changes that cause most of the diseases and conditions that plague living creatures as they grow old.' Rather than something to be ashamed of, our chronological age is a badge of honour, she adds. 'But the best, and perhaps only, way to truly earn more chronological years is by taking up arms against its unfortunate companion – biological age.' It can be made to tick faster or slower, according to our lifestyle. From a health perspective, if we could each slow ageing down by seven years, making a (chronological) seventy-year-old (biologically) sixty-three, their mortality risk from nearly every major disease would be cut in half, says Levine.

For the curious, nowadays we can have our spit analysed to ascertain our biological age, though simplistic online tests are available too (one said I was forty-one, though I'm paying more attention to my watch's calculation that I have the fitness age of a twenty-year-old).

Less scientifically, we also have a running age, namely how many years we've been regularly running for (making me thirteen). If you've come to the sport later in life, the great news is that even with a chronological age in the fifties or sixties, there's potentially huge performance and health progress to be made.

Runners aren't normal

Though it's discussed here, some or perhaps much of the science of ageing actually doesn't apply wholesale to us. Almost all of the research was carried out on people representative of society, a good proportion of whom are overweight, sedentary, exercise less often and/or have less healthy habits than runners. So the results of those studies aren't necessarily that instructive to us.

We know that even at a young age the worst diseases can already be developing in sedentary people, especially if they're not exercising or being conscious about lifestyle habits such as smoking or drinking. Much of what we know scientifically about ageing is based on these people. 'We didn't evolve for more than two million years to sit in front of the TV eating potato chips and contracting lifestyle diseases,' writes Joe Friel in *Fast After 50: How to Race Strong for the Rest of your Life*. 'Humans were meant to be active, to move vigorously and strenuously – just as you do as an athlete.' Compared to sedentary people around our age, we're biologically younger.

Even within sports science, there's a big question about how much of the research about 'active people' applies to committed amateur runners. 'They are comparing a wide range of abilities – from the front of the pack to the back – with not only physiology but also motivation playing a huge role,' writes Friel. 'Some people just aren't motivated to train and don't push themselves anywhere near their limits in a race.' This dilutes results, he argues, and we get better indicators of what age really does to us as runners by looking at the elite end (more anon).

And then so many studies are done on men, with the results clumsily and insultingly extrapolated to cover both sexes, when women have a very different health and fitness journey. We're still using lots of studies as guides to what's happening and what's possible for runners as we age, while knowing we may be, in some ways, beyond the science.

We runners are the normal ones. For our persistence-hunting ancestors, fitness was survival. It's not that what we know about ageing to date doesn't apply to us. Rather, we'll be affected by a smaller subset of symptoms. We're already outrunning the age pacer.

Seniors moment

We're at the forefront of a new frontier of longevity and sports science. Our parents weren't on Strava or getting out for three-hour runs at the weekend at our age. We're the first generation to be exercising in significant numbers well into our forties, fifties and beyond. We're not just exercising, but continuing to push for sporting excellence and age group PBs. The importance of exercise, alongside social booms in running, cycling, triathlon and other outdoor activities, plus so much more knowledge about anti-ageing, makes our generation performance pioneers. We're astronauts of ageing.

'We're virtual crash-test dummies for future generations who refuse to succumb to evolutionary stereotyping,' writes Phil Cavell in *The Midlife Cyclist: The Roadmap for the +40 Rider who Wants to Train Hard, Ride Fast and Stay Healthy*. 'This is a crucial time and we're the pathfinder generation for those that follow us.'

For example, in 2004 a man in his seventies beat the winning time of the first Olympic marathon. Ed Whitlock, a seventy-three-year-old Canadian, ran a record-setting 2:54:48 marathon, which beat the time of 2:58:50 set by twenty-three-year-old Spyridon Louis in Athens in 1896. So we're already pushing on further than before and the data we have may be a bit out of date anyway. It's an exciting time to be a masters athlete.

Running is health

As those gale-force winds of ageing batter our windows on this stormy night, let's gather around the small but hot fireplace of running and warm our hands a little. This is the perfect time to remind ourselves just how life-changingly incredible running is. 'If exercise was a pill, it would be prescribed to every patient' is one of the most quoted phrases – if not the most quoted phrase – in healthcare.

Running strengthens our heart, boosts respiratory function, lowers cholesterol and reduces risk of the worst diseases. Getting our daps on is good for our tendons, ligaments and joints. Despite popular legend, running won't wreck our knees. Instead, it actually strengthens them, with several studies suggesting recreational runners' joints are in better condition than non-runners'. Runners also have a significantly lower occurrence of osteoarthritis in the hips and knees compared to non-runners.

Elsewhere in the body, running rejuvenates mitochondria, the powerhouses of our cells, meaning muscle fibres can generate energy more efficiently. This is key, because our mitochondria become less effective as we age, but running stimulates their repair, allowing them to generate energy as efficiently as younger adults.

There's debate as to how much real strength running gives us. But there's no question that if someone's new to running, they'll experience strength gains in their lower limbs, increasing muscular power, strength, stability and balance.

Running is even linked to better sleep, better eye health and better cognitive health. Running is cheap, makes us feel great, enables quality 'me time', and gives us lifelong friends, community, memories, purpose and happiness. Running helps with body composition and weight loss (in one study, female runners gained 2 kilograms between the ages of twenty-nine and sixty, while non-runners gained 9 kilograms). It's a way to explore, have adventures, take on challenges, surprise ourselves, accomplish difficult things, boost self-esteem and feel better about ourselves. We don't need scientists to tell us running is really, really good for us in so many ways. Runners know it.

Running is mental health

Running gives us huge mental health benefits. Ever felt more relaxed and energised after a run? Jogging is repeatedly cited as helpful to lift mental loads and reduce feelings of stress and anxiety. Research found that running therapy and antidepressants had similar effects on the mental health of patients with depression and/or anxiety disorder, while a small study found that even a relatively short bout of exercise led to a 58% reduction in cognitive stress.

It'll be no surprise that running in green places has even more mental health benefits. People who exercise in nature experience increased energy levels and decreased feelings of depression and are more likely to repeat their workouts. Indeed, 89% of parkrun participants said that running regularly made them feel happier and had a positive impact on their mental health. Numerous studies connect nature to well-being and biophilia, our innate desire to be in nature.

Runners are smarter

Running also has huge psychological benefits. It makes us smarter. There is insurmountable evidence that regular exercise helps to curb age-related mental decline, found a study.[2] Adults over the age of fifty who take up aerobic exercise benefit from better cognitive function. Scientists had never understood the curious ability of exercise to boost brain power, but in 2010 Cambridge University scientists proved that running stimulates the brain to grow fresh grey matter.[3] A few days of running led to the growth of hundreds of thousands of new brain cells that improved the ability to recall memories without confusing them. The new brain cells appeared in a region linked to the formation and recollection of memories, the hippocampus.

So, running can improve memory and learning – and potentially slow the deterioration of mental ability that happens with ageing. Scientists are unsure why exactly exercise triggers the growth of grey matter, but it may be linked to increased blood flow or higher levels of hormones released while exercising. Studies have found running can help with your decision-making abilities, and that high-intensity exercises can assist adolescents with focus and problem-solving. Runners literally have a 'younger-appearing brain', concluded one study.

Running can change the brain in many of the same ways that activities requiring fine motor skills do, like playing an instrument or a racquet sport – which have also been strongly linked to longevity in studies, with perhaps greater effect (probably due to the extra mental component). Conventional logic says that running isn't mentally taxing. Just repeatedly put one foot in front of the other and try not to trip on a shoelace. But running was found to be a pretty cognitively demanding sport. The root in the trail, the traffic light about to turn red and the non-attentive dog owner are all challenges we have to navigate on a second-by-second basis. 'As hunter-gatherers, we moved quickly around the landscape, but we'd also have to remember where we were going, use spatial navigation, and executive functions like planning and decision-making,' says Professor David Raichlen, an anthropologist who studies runners and the evolutionary history of exercise. 'We think those cognitive skills got linked to exercise through evolutionary processes.'

Skeleton grew

We know that bone health deteriorates as we age, but there's some relatively good news for runners. When used, our muscles pull on our bones, sending signals that encourage new bone formation, so weight-bearing exercise helps. However, while our sport is more beneficial than non-weight-bearing exercises such as cycling or swimming, easy running isn't enough to stimulate significant new growth. A study comparing endurance runners to the sedentary detected barely any difference in bone health. Sprinters, however, had 14% higher bone density. So the faster we run and the higher the impact, the better it is for bone health. That said, an Italian study found that ultramarathon runners had higher P1NP levels – an indication of bone health – compared to the control group. So perhaps longer runs create relevant amounts of force, too?

Strength training has an even better impact. Lifting three times a week leads to a 3% increase in bone density over a year, found a study in which those who didn't lift lost 1%. Resistance training also helps keep our tendons strong because they thrive on being loaded. (The calf–Achilles complex is a key one for runners to work on.)

Running away from death

Research into more than 55,000 people showed that those who run for 1–3 hours per week have a 30% lower risk of death.[4] Just ten minutes a day reduces all-cause mortality and death from cardiovascular disease, specifically by improving the health of our cells, which in turn fight off ageing. Running doesn't just extend lifespan, it could greatly improve our health-span, the idea of remaining healthy for longer. Few of us would choose to live to 100 if it meant a decade or two of slowly dying in a chair, and myriad studies have attested to exercise's ability to reduce the chances of a visit from the Four Horsemen. Indeed, when it comes to disease resistance, running is queen. Pounding the pavements (other surfaces are available) helps to boost our respiratory function, hugely lower our cholesterol, and reduce our risk of diabetes and cardiovascular disease. There are so many studies with these types of results.

While running doesn't cure cancer, it can help to prevent it. If you run regularly, you may have a 70% lower risk of developing colon cancer, 30–40% less chance of developing breast cancer and (although results here were less clear) a reduction in the overall risk of prostate cancer ranging from 5% to 65%. Running three times a week for an average of just seventeen minutes at a time reduced the risk of fatal heart attack or stroke by as much as 50%, found a large study.[5] For some, regular aerobic exercise is part of a successful treatment plan for cancer.

Though there is no known effective treatment to prevent or stop the progression of Alzheimer's, running gives us a much greater chance of dodging it. A study of women who were highly fit in their forties to their sixties found that their risk of dementia decreased by nearly 90%.[6] In a study of 649,000 US (male) masters with an average age of sixty-one, the fittest in the group were 33% less likely to develop Alzheimer's after nine years than the least fit.[7]

The findings suggest that the association between cardiorespiratory fitness and Alzheimer's risk is inverse: the fitter you are, the less likely you may be to get Alzheimer's. Another study found that brain inflammation reduces by 55–68% in those who exercise regularly.[8] Although this evidence – and much of the existing research – is currently limited to animal studies, it still suggests that aerobic exercise has the potential to significantly reduce disease markers associated with Alzheimer's.

In fact, running was probably key to allowing *Homo sapiens* to reach old age in the first place. Thousands of years ago, our ancestors had two copies of a genotype that greatly increases the risk of Alzheimer's and cardiovascular disease. However, humans began living much longer than other mammals at this time. Professor David Raichlen believes that the need to constantly be on the move – in order to find food and to run from danger – caused our hearts to enlarge and our capillaries to grow. This minimised the chances of developing these diseases, despite the presence of the high-risk genes. 'I tend to think that exercise explains quite a bit about why we are the way we are today,' Raichlen says, pointing out that our risk of chronic disease has surged as our time spent exercising has plummeted. By not running, we're negating or even reversing our evolutionary history.[9]

Running pushes back against senescence and makes us healthier in many ways. As we age, our arteries stiffen and can't widen as well as they used to in order to accommodate an increase in blood flow, particularly in the aorta (the artery leading from the heart) and the carotid arteries (which run from the chest to the head). When this happens, major cardiac events aren't far behind. But aerobic exercise restores elasticity and dilation to arteries, allowing them to behave years younger, while restoring youth and vigour to the vessels.

Run one step and all our muscles – quads, calves, glutes, even our lats, shoulders and biceps – demand more oxygen. To feed them, we suck in air, our heart beats faster and it pumps oxygenated blood through the arteries to every muscle fibre. The process isn't just a delivery mechanism. It's invisibly keeping our arteries strong and healthy, transforming our heart into a younger version of itself. When arteries are healthy, science shows that everything outside the cardiovascular system is usually healthy, too. Cognitive decline and disease are closely linked to deterioration in artery function and health. The increased risk of diabetes as we age is highly correlated with vascular health and function. Kidney disease is also closely linked to the health of our arteries, as are neurodegenerative diseases and inflammation. It's scary stuff. But much less so if we're runners. **We joggers can slash our risk of cardiovascular-related death – the world's biggest killer – by 45–70%.**

Regardless of how old you are, whether you're male or female, how much booze you drink or whether you've ever exercised before, if you start running just 1–2 hours per week, it can dramatically increase your odds of living longer.

Running also strengthens lungs, helps to regulate blood sugar and therefore manage body weight, and strengthens the immune system – ever notice you don't get viruses as often as your non-runner friends? For anyone over sixty, working out once or twice a week reduces all-cause mortality by 50% and reduces the risk of cancer threefold. 'Motion is lotion' and 'mobility is medicine' are other popular healthcare mantras.

In short, keep running and you can increase both the quantity and quality of your years.

Ageless aces

If you needed any more convincing, just wait till you hear about this lot. We're already seeing a new wave of senescence fighters kicking age's butt.

Just a quick reality check, though: generally, elite sportspeople are in their prime between the disgustingly young ages of twenty and thirty. Indeed, 90% of competitors at the 2021 Tokyo Olympics were under thirty, the youngest being just twelve years old.

In running, female marathoners peak at twenty-nine and male runners at twenty-seven, according to a study of the top ten runners in each five-year age group at the New York Marathon. The window of physical and sporting excellence may feel depressingly short and a long time ago; the fact most of us probably weren't conscious we were in our physical prime at the time adds to the nostalgia (at that age I was keener to chase down beer than PBs).

In elite sport, following that peak there's a slow physiological decline that's hardly perceptible at first and can be masked by the advantages of experience and small changes in training, meaning that small performance gains are still possible. 'In fact, it may be attributed to poor training, minor changes in lifestyle, or even bad luck,' writes TrainingPeaks founder and *Fast After 50* author Joe Friel, albeit 'by the early forties it's generally obvious to most high-performance athletes that things are going the wrong direction.'

In football, the world's most popular sport, most players are done at the very top level by their early thirties. The decline is so sharp that they are almost all playing at a lower standard or less frequently by thirty-five and traditionally almost all retired by their fortieth birthday. Traditionally.

However, more recently we've seen numerous glorious masters not just surviving at the very top of elite sport in their forties, but winning. Tom Brady was the NFL's Most Valuable Player (MVP) at forty, the Super Bowl MVP at forty-three and selected to the Pro Bowl at forty-four (all the oldest on record). Meanwhile, in the NHL, ice hockey player Jaromír Jágr was still leading the Florida Panthers and still scoring aged forty-four. Cyclist Kristin Armstrong didn't win her first Olympic gold till she was thirty-five, and went on to win her third gold at the 2016 Rio Games the day before her forty-third birthday. In tennis, Serena Williams was winning titles well into her late thirties, while Roger Federer was winning them in his forties. Tiger Woods and Jack Nicklaus did the same in golf. Football superstar Cristiano Ronaldo is still playing and scoring on the big stage as I write, aged forty. In surfing, Kelly Slater is still winning prestigious competitions aged fifty.

These aren't outliers. Something is happening. The number of NBA players aged thirty-five or over jumped from two to thirty-two between 1982 and 2015. In the NHL, it's gone from four to fifty over the same period; in the NFL, from fourteen to thirty-eight. The average age of the top ten men in tennis has increased by five years since 1992. 'In virtually every sport, athletes are sticking around for an extra victory lap or three rather than shuffling off to the metaphorical showers at the first sign of gray,' writes Jeff Bercovici in *Play On: The New Science of Elite Performance at Any Age*.

'Masters athletes remain a fascinating model of "exceptionally successful ageing" and are therefore deserving of our continued scientific attention as physiologists', concluded one study.[10] 'A revolution is happening in endurance sports,' agrees renowned US sports writer and author Matt Fitzgerald. 'Athletes over the age of fifty are breaking records at an unprecedented rate, performing at levels that were unimaginable ten years ago.'[11]

In elite road and track running, Britain's Jo Pavey (more on page 44) is the oldest European champion in history, claiming a 10,000 metres gold aged forty and competing at the Olympics aged forty-two. The US's Sara Hall ran an American masters marathon record of 2:23:45 aged forty-one, while her compatriot Meb Keflezighi won the Boston Marathon two weeks before his thirty-ninth birthday, making him the oldest winner since 1930. In October 2025, forty-two-year-old Maria Lindberg, a cancer survivor and mother of three, became the first masters athlete to hit the qualifying time for the US Olympic Marathon Trials. She ran 2:34:59, bettering her PB by almost fifteen minutes. Nearly half of the records for events longer than 800 metres and for ages fifty-plus have been set since 2020.

'Younger athletes are getting faster too, but older athletes are getting faster more quickly,' writes Matt Fitzgerald. He reports that at the World Triathlon Age-Group Championships, the 2014 winner of the women's 60–64 division finished 22:18 behind the winner of the 30–34 division. Ten years later, the gap was down to 17:14; and on the men's side, the gap shrank from 18:24 to 13:23.

In endurance sports, such as running, swimming, cycling and triathlon, the decline is initially so slight that it may not even be noticed, especially compared to sports based on power, speed and fast-twitch fibres. In ultramarathon running, where admittedly top-end speed is less of a factor but still not insignificant, France's evergreen Ludovic Pommeret set a course record at the prestigious Hardrock 100 (10,000 metres of elevation gain, reaching 4,280 metres in height) at the age of forty-nine, beating the record previously held by the much younger GOAT Kílian Jornet. Meanwhile, over here Nicky Spinks is still winning races at fifty-eight (see page 83). Jasmin Paris was forty when she made history by being the first female finisher of the infamous Barkley Marathons. Harita Davies won the Self-Transcendence 3100 Mile Race in 2021, aged forty-five. Marianne Heading won the Montane Yukon Arctic Ultra outright, aged forty-seven. Florence Golay-Geymond set a new course record for the 450-kilometre Tor des Glaciers, aged fifty-two. There isn't space to dive fully into it here, but there's plenty of anecdotal and a little bit of scientific evidence to suggest midlife females are especially strong at longer distances.

Indeed, ultramarathon PBs are generally achieved at the age of thirty-five to forty-five or older, for both women and men, and the age of peak performance increases with the race distance or duration.

Winners of Ironman triathlons are getting older, with similar trends for elite ultramarathoners, noted a 2016 study.[12] During the four decades to 2009, the age of the top five runners at the prestigious Western States Endurance Run increased from the early to the upper thirties. Other ultras are frequently won by runners in their forties. Researchers commented that, 'These data show that the upper age limit of elite ultra-endurance athletes has increased during the past decades, bringing into question what the upper limit of the age of peak performance in elite ultra-endurance performance actually is.'

The age-related decline in ultra-endurance performance ranges from 8% to 15% per decade with advancing age, according to a study on the 100-kilometre distance. Yet the increase in participation of masters athletes in ultra events has been accompanied by an improvement in their performance at a faster rate than young athletes.

In sub-elite sport, the trend for age-defying performances and simply more people having a go is clear. Participation in the World Masters Games has tripled since 1985, with the 2017 edition featuring 25,000 athletes over forty. The standard graph of age-related performance decline can be significantly different for recreational runners, especially if we sign up to Strava later in life. Indeed, middle-aged runners consistently average faster marathon times than their younger rivals, according to a Strava study – though that's likely down to lifestyle and motivation factors more than physiological (more anon).

Also, those who come to running later in life, and train hard and consistently, can still run their quickest marathons in their forties, fifties and sixties. Just look at the example of Belgium's Jo Schoonbroodt, who set a marathon world record for the V70 category in 2022. His time? 2:54:19. All around us, seniors are doing sensational things. At the 5K distance the age-category world records look like this:

Age group	Women	Men
V40	15:43	13:38
V50	16:38	15:00
V60	18:13	16:06
V70	21:17	17:59
V80	24:08	22:41
V90	46:24	33:46

Right up to the V70 age category, many fit twenty-year-olds would struggle to get near those times. While we have to acknowledge that we will experience some level of performance decline by the age of fifty, it could be smaller than we might imagine. A study of track athletes aged fifty to eighty-five found a decline of less than 2% between the ages of fifty and seventy-five. It wasn't until seventy-five that performance in events ranging from 100 metres to 10,000 metres started to fall by about 8% per year.

'I think my time away from serious running has helped my longevity now.'

TOMMY HUGHES

Tommy, sixty-five, ran the marathon for Ireland at the 1992 Olympics in Barcelona, after a PB of 2:13:15 at the Marrakech Marathon. Aged thirty-two, the electrician then took a sixteen-year-break from the sport (more on page 33), returning at forty-eight. In 2019, aged fifty-nine, he ran the Frankfurt Marathon in a new world record time for his age of 2:27:52. That run is also part of a record for the fastest father–son marathon, with his son, Eoin, running 2:31:30 for a combined time of 4:59:22. In 2020, aged sixty, Tommy set a new world record for the half marathon of 1:11:09 – which WAVA says is an age-grading equivalent to 57:47. He also set another marathon record that year, with 2:30:02, breaking the previous age-group record by over 6 minutes. The Irishman also holds the V60 world record for 5,000 metres, with 16:47.59. The ageless ace's Instagram handle makes his current goals clear: @breaking2.30at60

When I ran in the Olympics in Barcelona, it was very hot. Four years later, the Olympics was going to be in Atlanta and I decided not to even try. It was going to be very hard again and I just hadn't the incentive. It's either all or nothing with me. So I went all-in for work, trying to make as much money as I could.

I'm an electrician. I was working away from home a lot, in southern Ireland, England, Scotland, Saudi Arabia, China. I just didn't have the time to train. I would still run, on and off, but I wasn't consistent. Anything needs to be consistent if you want to be good at it. I always felt I had a natural ability in running, because I could come back quick, from being out of shape to running pretty fast. So it never bothered me to take a break.

The Belfast Marathon brought me back to running. I had won it in 1988 and 1998. It was 2008 and I had the idea of winning it again. But the Kenyans were there and I ended up sixth. I looked around after that and there were the V50 world records. I could go for those.

I work hard at anything I do. I was just off, you know, going at it, being consistent. It takes me two to three months, usually, of dedication to get properly fit. I'd got it up in the head that I wanted to get quicker and quicker, to try to break the age category records. And that's what I've done.

I think my time away from serious running has helped my longevity now. I think you get burned out very quickly if you keep going hard at something for a long time. Mentally, you get burned out. Or, physically, your body starts to break down. So any breaks in between, there's no harm at all.

My long run at the weekend is usually about 23 miles, or the occasional marathon distance. Most of my training is steady running. I was up to 130 miles a week and I was getting fitter and fitter, just because I was doing the miles. Your body becomes attuned to it. I've always trained on my own. I just get my gear on and I'm away out the door.

I do two runs a day. In the morning I might do about seven miles or so; in the evening I might do nine. I don't do intervals as such. Races are my tempos, doing 10Ks and half marathons when I fancy, you know, to get the legs turning over a lot quicker. You put more effort into races than doing intervals on your own.

I don't have a rest day every week. But I do listen to my body and if I think I'm doing too much, I just take a rest day. I used to train hard and work hard and not get anywhere. Because I wasn't resting.

The only strength work I do is some press-ups. My diet's not that strict, but I try to eat healthy, to get all the vitamins and nutrients. I'm not a believer in taking any supplements or anything. Everybody's got their own way of doing it and I just judge for myself what I need to do, not what anybody else tells me to do. It's worked for me for all my life. I have a very strong mental side. If I put my mind to something, I will go for it.

For marathons, age is a big advantage. That's where age is a good balancer. If you prepare right, you can beat a younger guy, because if they don't prepare right, you're going to beat them. You lose your speed getting older, but the stamina is still there. That's why the marathon has always been a good leveller and older runners can benefit; they've got the stamina and the mental fortitude. That's all you need.

I've known people that raced really well when they were younger, came to a certain age and they're going, 'Well, I can't do what I've done before, so I'm not doing it at all.' But I enjoy competing against the younger ones a lot. I'm getting slower and that's just the way it is. Maybe it will come to a time when I'll say, forget about racing and just enjoy staying fit, going out and not hammering yourself all the time.

If I can't run competitively any more, I can just run for fun. That definitely wouldn't bother me too much at all. I don't have to prove anything to anybody. I do this for my own enjoyment. I've done more than I ever thought I could do. If somebody told me that I'd be going to the Olympics, I wouldn't have believed them. No way. So to get to do that, I was so over the moon. And from then on everything else was a bonus.

To midlife runners I'd say, just go out and enjoy your run. Enjoy your company. If you run with other people, enjoy their company. Enjoy your running. That's all you need to do. Some people get too wound up about competing.

That said, I still believe 2:30 is breakable for me. I can do it. I'm sixty-six in January 2026 and I will be retirement age, so the government will be paying me to be a full-time runner at last!

Prime plus

The rate of athletic decline is actually reassuringly slow. Because distance running is more endurance-based than most sports, and therefore initially less affected by ageing, runners actually slide from their peak later and fairly slowly. Meanwhile, sports with speed and power – which prioritise fast-twitch fibres over distance-running's slower twitch fibres – fade sooner, as those fibres switch from speed to endurance. So what does that decline look like for distance runners?

While performance can decrease from thirty years old, a study found that, 'Peak endurance performance is maintained until about thirty-five years of age, followed by modest decreases until fifty to sixty years of age, with progressively steeper declines thereafter.'[13] Other studies suggest another drop-off after seventy.

Rather than being a slow and steady process, ageing may occur in at least two accelerated bursts. This idea of an ageing cliff, a sudden drop in health or overnight increase in wrinkles, is debated. Some research shows that athletically we may fall or stumble down a cliff in our fifties and again in our seventies. As mentioned earlier, 2024 Stanford research into the general population suggested cliffs around the age of forty-four and again around sixty. That's not just linked to menopause, but it seems to happen in men too, according to the study, which tracked thousands of molecules in 108 people aged twenty-five to seventy-five. The first wave of changes included molecules linked to cardiovascular disease and the ability to metabolise caffeine, alcohol and lipids. The second wave included molecules involved in immune regulation, carbohydrate metabolism and kidney function. Molecules linked to skin and muscle ageing changed at both time points.[14]

It may be that the cliffs that occur in sedentary people in their forties and sixties happen to runners later, in their fifties and seventies. Either way, runners' marathon times are 2% slower for every year after their late-twenties peak. So a woman who runs a 3:00:00 marathon aged twenty-nine is capable of 3:02:36 the following year; while a twenty-seven-year-old man who runs a 3:30:00 marathon, if he maintains peak training, is capable of clocking 3:34:12 a year later. This assumes they were both at their peak at those ages, both physiologically and in training.

But wait – another study has even better news. Between thirty-five and forty, runners slowed down by only 1% over the five-year span. A 2018 Yale University study looked at 5K, 10K, half marathon and marathon results from 200 male (hmm!) runners aged forty to ninety-five who'd set world records in their respective age groups.[15]

'You don't see any real fitness declines until age forty,' said Dr Ray Fair. The study found that between the ages of forty and seventy, runners slowed by a linear rate of about 1% each year or 10% per decade, until they reached their late seventies, when they began to decline by about 1.5%; between ninety and ninety-five, that rate accelerated to a 2–3% decline. 'Even at age ninety, people are only a little more than twice as slow as they were in their peak years,' Fair told *Runner's World*.

But not all studies take into account changes in lifestyle, motivation levels, injury and other factors. A slight decline in VO2 max may be offset by the ability to deal with greater amounts of lactic acid, an advantage found in older runners. This could explain why many endurance athletes in their late forties and fifties are able to remain competitive with athletes in their twenties and thirties. In the 2012 Boston Marathon, the winner of the male 40–44 age-category ran 2:23:08, finishing in fifteenth place just 10:28 behind the overall winner. In Ironman events, the top finishers aged 40–50 consistently place in the top twenty to fifty overall, out of thousands of participants.

Tommy Hughes (previous pages) will cheer you up. In 2019, the fifty-nine-year-old Irishman ran a jaw-dropping 2:27 marathon. Hughes's VO2 max was 65.4, more than twice what you'd expect from a largely sedentary man his age. But Hughes is a former Olympic marathoner who had taken a sixteen-year break, starting again at the age of forty-eight. If that break did hurt him, it wasn't by much. He currently holds the world marathon record for the 60–64 age group, at 2:30:02.

Elsewhere, Hans Smeets is a seventy-five-year-old middle-distance runner who holds multiple European and world age-group records, with a VO2 max of 50.5, equal to the highest known measurement for his age. Smeets only began running at fifty, and over the next twenty-five years he never missed more than a week of training. Initially, he ran more than

85 miles per week, and at seventy-five he was still logging 50 miles. He attributed his ability to train so consistently without injury to running at 'an easy pace'. Smeets and Hughes have huge VO_2 max scores and are clearly outliers, so does their late-age excellence really tell us much?

The conventional view had been that as you get older, the decline gets steeper, with a 'break point' sometime after seventy. But recent research into the role of lifelong endurance exercise as a countermeasure against age-related decline in VO_2 max correlated scores across different ages and found no evidence that VO_2 max values fall off a cliff beyond a certain point. This suggests that **the steepest declines probably happen when you start exercising less, rather than as a result of hitting a particular age**. 'You don't train less because you're getting old,' says *Endure* author and sports-science journalist Alex Hutchinson. 'You get old, to a surprising extent, because skipping that long Sunday run with your pals becomes a habit instead of a rare exception. Don't do it.' This feels like excellent news.

Frustratingly, however, that study was on men and there may be some gender differences. Statistically, female runners decline a little faster than males. There's a 20% difference between male and female finishing times until the age of fifty-five, when the gap starts to widen. By the age of seventy, women are about 40% slower than men. But that finding may be influenced by a small study-pool size.

As well as indicating our athletic capabilities, our VO_2 max can inform how long we will live and how functional we will be in later years, and our VO_2 max is probably a better indicator of our body's health status than our chronological age, says Joe Friel.

As we age, we know our athletic potential declines. But our ability to maximise our potential doesn't.

These may be outliers and we're talking more simply about doing very difficult things at ages when most people don't, rather than about optimal performance, but as I was researching this book, Natalie Grabow became the oldest woman to complete an Ironman, aged eighty, in 16 hours and 45 minutes. Meanwhile, eighty-year-old Bob Becker finished Badwater, a 135-mile ultramarathon through California's sweltering Death Valley. At seventy, he became the oldest person to complete the 'Badwater Double'

– turning around to run back to the race start after completing the official 135-mile event.

Nurture over nature

Ageing is not genetic. This feels huge. **Ageing is much more nurture than nature.** Senescence isn't the only factor in athletic decline. In midlife we might have children, which, while indisputably wonderful, affects sleep, finances and availability to train. Work might ask more of us, sleep and diet might suffer, training might take a hit, and performances likewise, which affects our motivation. And we're in an athletic-ageing doom spiral. Perhaps we get a motivation bump post-Christmas or after watching the London Marathon and we jump excitedly back into training. And get injured. Meaning a break from training and more decline. So how much of the ageing process is an inevitable physical fade and how much is a result of lifestyle and consistent quality training not always being the happiest bedfellows?

Renowned triathlon coach Alan Couzens noticed a pleasing symmetry in data from his athletes. All else being equal, the amount of aerobic fitness lost by getting a year older was almost identical to the amount gained by adding an hour per month of training time. So in theory, freezing the biological clock from one birthday merely required an additional fifteen minutes per week of running. This may sound simple, but after a decade that additional training time would total 2.5 hours a week, not to mention our increased susceptibility to injury and the double demons of lifestyle and motivation. So the reality and wisdom of that approach is debatable. And VO2 max will still decline.

Around 50% of the fitness losses suffered by endurance athletes as they get older are attributable to the passage of time, found research which pooled the results of more than a dozen studies. The other half can be explained by reduced training. Joe Friel speculates the balance could be as much as 60:40 or even 70:30. Whatever the exact equation is, the idea is huge.

How we age is 70–90% down to us, our lifestyle and the decisions we make, according to a study of over 20,000 Danish, Finnish and Swedish twins.[16] We're not prisoners of our genes and our DNA, which only account for 10–30% of how we age anyway. Sporting and health longevity is in our hands.

Women are not small men

Women and men are not the same. We have crucially different physiologies. Until recently, research into female athletes ranged from limited to non-existent, with female athletes often being treated as small men. Dr Stacy Sims, aged fifty-one and the author of *Roar* and *Next Level,* is rebalancing science's sexism by pioneering research in exercise nutrition and performance, focused on women. Her books are essential reading and it's worth seeking her out on podcasts. That women have a menstrual cycle and experience menopause should have made it blindingly obvious that our bodies are different, but for ages sports science treated men and women the same. Menopause is discussed by Renee McGregor on page 48. But what are the other key differences?

Women are born with more oxidative fibres than men (who have more glycolytic/anaerobic fibres), so they already have really robust mitochondria, mitochondrial function and mitochondrial respiration. That means greater metabolic flexibility and greater ability for burning free fatty acids. Women's bodies default when they're in low energy to burn fat preferentially (whereas men go through their blood sugars first, then liver glycogen, then muscle glycogen stores, all before they get into fat burning).

From a training standpoint, male runners need to include more low-intensity, zone 2 work to gain that metabolical flexibility and tap into burning more body fat. 'Women are already super endurance,' explains Sims. '[Oestrogen's] components encourage sparing carbohydrate and encourage the use of free fatty acids, so there's another layer [...] that allow[s] women to be very successful at endurance.'

Women need to rethink volume, she argues. 'We need time on the feet, but we don't need to do the significant amount of volume that's ingrained in all of the running programs, because those are all based on male data.' Women need to do 'intensity across the board' to teach the brain and the muscles how to use that high intensity, plus one-legged exercises for control, stability and overall running technique.

Men over fifty may have to exercise more than twice as much as women to get the same heart health benefits, a 2025 study found.[17] So there are some sex differences that are only just being uncovered.

Women need different fuelling, too. Women have more gastrointestinal (GI) distress (attributable to gastrointestinal transit time, sensitivity, and the specific effects of oestrogen and progesterone on gut function). During performance, they need more mixed and macronutrient food and some carbohydrates, rather than the quick hits of simple sugar or gels. Their gut can't handle as much fructose or maltodextrin as men.

Women also respond differently to heat and cold stresses. But the key thing is that men and women are different, and to date most science is based on men.

Running forever

Notwithstanding the fact barflies will always need convincing that running doesn't in fact lead directly to arthritic knees or heart attacks (more anon), it'll come as little surprise that runners live longer.

Indeed, **elite runners live for years longer than non-runners**, a study released on the seventieth anniversary of Sir Roger Bannister's sub-four-minute mile record revealed.[18] Researchers in Canada and Australia tracked down the health records of the first 200 people to complete a sub-four-minute mile, including runners from the UK, Australia, France, New Zealand and the United States who were born between 1928 and 1955. All 200 runners were men. The study's authors not only noted that the runners lived on average almost five years longer than the general population, but they also analysed how healthy their lives were by accessing their medical records. Just sixty of the runners had died. 'We know that elite athletes have bigger hearts due to their sustained aerobic output and there was some belief that this could affect their health and longevity,' said Professor André La Gerche. 'Five years of extra life compared to average is very significant, especially when we found that many of these runners not only enjoyed long lives but were also healthy. Not everyone needs to be able to run a sub-four-minute mile to enjoy good health long into old age, but they need to exercise regularly and push themselves aerobically.'

Tell the barflies that.

Running may even add nineteen years to our lives, concluded a study of serious marathon runners.[19] Ben Rosin, a long-time American marathoner, cardiologist and cardiac rehab specialist, noted how his old training partners in their seventies and eighties seemed to be holding up well. So he analysed fifty-four of his friends who'd run numerous marathons against the general population and discovered his running pals were living, on average, nineteen years longer than US men who reached the age of forty in 1975 at about the same time as them.

For balance, it wasn't a controlled trial and other fitness and longevity studies have found less life extension. For example, a study of Tour de France riders gave them an eight-year advantage over gen pop, while other research has generally concluded that modest and high fitness is worth an extra three to eight years of life.

Outrunning ageing

This is the big one: running makes us younger. Yes, it may not feel like it 18 miles into a marathon-specific long run or again when we look in the mirror the next morning to see a wrinkly, half-awake face staring back. But science indubitably says it does. **Getting our daps on has a unique anti-ageing effect on our cells and can add twelve years to our life**, even on as little as 75 minutes per week, according to a 2023 study. The research looked at more than 4,400 subjects, comparing those who ran at least 75 minutes a week with those who ran less than 10 minutes a week. They found that the difference equated to 'roughly a twelve-year cellular ageing advantage associated with jogging/running'.[20]

The study examined telomeres, structures found at the end of chromosomes. The longer and more numerous they are, the better our cellular health. As we age, their quantity and length decrease, but exercise can help to slow the decline.

Another study verified that three 45-minute running sessions per week led to stronger telomeres, which help us age better, with stronger cardiac and muscular function.[21] The more your telomeres stay intact, the more resistant the cells are to stress and inflammation. Again, the study was on inactive people, so runners are accidentally already benefitting from anti-ageing tactics.

Researchers at Brigham Young University wanted to explore how physical activity influences ageing at the cellular level. Their study focused on telomeres.[22] The researchers discovered that adults who ran for 30–40 minutes per day (or did equivalent physical activity), five days per week had significantly longer telomeres than less active individuals. In fact, people who maintained a high level of physical activity had a biological advantage of approximately nine years compared to those who were sedentary. In simple terms, **active adults – especially runners – show cellular markers of youthfulness nearly a decade younger than their inactive peers.**

Another study showed that young sedentary people had telomeres 16% longer than old sedentary people.[23] But comparing young with old groups of endurance-trained people found just a 7% difference. 'Telomeres are the best-known markers of our cell age and their length is directly correlated to our activity levels,' said the study. Scientists can't explain exactly why, but exercise slows ageing by keeping our telomeres young.

A 2018 study found that seventy-five-year-olds who did about seven hours a week of aerobic exercise (running, swimming or cycling) over the course of their lives had similar cardiovascular health to a typical forty-five-year-old.[24] A 2020 study on first-time marathoners discovered that averaging just 6–13 miles a week decreased the stiffness in participants' arteries, equivalent to a reversal in the age of their vascular system of about four years.[25] The training also lowered their systolic blood pressure, and therefore their risk of stroke, by approximately 10% over the course of their life. Numerous studies have shown this.

It gets better. Middle-aged hearts can regain youthful power in just two years of structured exercise, found a recent study. Researchers at UT Southwestern enrolled sixty-one previously sedentary adults and found that four to five weekly sessions effectively rewound heart age by twenty years. The regimen mixed recreational 'base pace' workouts with interval bursts, peaking at six hours a week. Again, runners are already benefitting from this.

Running isn't just fantastic for us – regular exercise is the very best thing we can do to combat senescence. Tell your non-runner pals that even going from zero exercise per week to 90 minutes is predicted to reduce their risk of dying by 14%. Study after study has found that **regular exercisers live as much as a decade longer than sedentary people. They also stay in better health, with less morbidity** (suffering from disease or a medical condition) from causes related to metabolic dysfunction. We know you'll have more energy too, to enjoy life more.

The age advantage

Seniority is an athletic advantage. I was dubious at first, but in ultra-marathons previous experience – i.e. the number of previous finishes – is a greater predictor of success than training measures, found a study.

'Wisdom cancels out some of the advantages of youth,' insists sports coach Chris Carmichael. 'If young athletes behaved like older athletes, they could be even stronger and faster. Remember the old adage that youth is wasted on the young? It's generally true in endurance sports. Older athletes tend to have the means and patience to eat fresher and more nutrient-dense foods. They're more willing to go to bed earlier if their coaches tell them they need more rest. Many older athletes are more comfortable with their career and family lives, which translates to lower levels of lifestyle stress. And older athletes know themselves better, have more confidence, and are often better at listening to the signals their bodies are sending them. In other words, age gives some people the wisdom to be better at being athletes.'

Mature athletes have a much stronger sense of perspective, says sports psychologist Dr Josephine Perry. 'It's just running, right? I see fourteen-, fifteen-year-olds throwing up before competitions because they're so anxious about the outcome and what it means about them as a person. Forty-year-olds are like, "Okay, it's just a run. Let's have fun." That's a much better place to be. Because you've lived through so much, you've got perspective of what really matters.'

Perry cites 2025 Winter Spine Race winner Lucy Gossage as an 'amazing example' of this. 'Her first Winter Spine Race was all about doing it alongside a partner and the two of them having been on this whole journey from doing their first ultra to kind of going to do the ultimate ultra, the 2024 Winter Spine Race. Then she found out he was a total fraud and had to get her head around that, which is a big ask. She stood on the start line in 2025, and "the start line became my finish line," she said, "because I'm standing on the start line and realising, I've processed it all now. Now I'm here for me." That sense of perspective she had, I imagine, got her through some of those really, really difficult times in the Spine.'

Mature athletes can use life experience to take away a lot of the pressure and the expectation and go just to run. **The run just doesn't matter as much.** 'A run doesn't impact whether I'm a good or bad person,' says Perry. 'Our identity is less wrapped in a particular run or in running. We've developed less of a mono identity.'

As well as perspective, purpose and life experience, crucially we've also built up reams of performance experience. 'You can't surprise me on defence,' Tom Brady said in an interview shortly after winning a record fifth Super Bowl at thirty-nine. 'I've seen it all. I've processed 261 games, I've played them all. It's an incredibly hard sport, but because the processes are right and are in place, for anyone with experience in their job, it's not as hard as it used to be. There was a time when quarterbacking was really hard for me, because you didn't know what to do. Now I really know what to do.'

As athletes accumulate experience within their sports, they become more efficient processors of information, writes Jeff Bercovici in *Play On*. 'The longer you play, the faster you think.' While running may seem like a simpler sport on the surface, when trails are involved – plus fuelling, hydration, even sleeping, pacing and motivation strategies for the really long ones – there is a great deal to think about and it's not such a huge surprise that older athletes do so well. 'At fifty-five, it is difficult to win shorter races, but in ultrarunning races where you have to be able to strategise, problem-solve, run and endure, age and experience can outweigh speed,' said Anna Troup after her 2025 overall win at the 268-mile Summer Spine Race.

It's about patience, says Alex Hutchinson: 'When you're older, you can see the bigger picture more than you could when you were seventeen. We have patience. It's really easy to get excited about big goals, but to actually achieve them requires patience to take care of details, patience to stay on track when obstacles arise. Older people are more patient.'

As humans, we possess both fluid and crystallised intelligence. Fluid intelligence relates to short-term memory, but crystallised intelligence uses learnings accumulated over a lifespan and is thought to increase through our sixties and seventies.

In *The Attributes: 25 Hidden Drivers of Optimal Performance,* former Navy SEAL Rich Diviney identifies discipline, resilience, open-mindedness and humour as sometimes better indicators than skill as to whether someone might stumble or succeed at arduous endeavours. These are all attributes we'd more commonly associate with experienced athletes.

Also, perhaps because of some of those things, we're likely to just be happier. That's the pattern detected in many large-scale studies. In general, people start off with a high degree of contentment. From around the age of eighteen, our happiness gradually declines, reaching a nadir in our forties. However, as we enter our fifties, levels of contentment climb again and reach new highs in our sixties. This U-shaped curve is consistently clear in data from American and European studies. We're talking averages here, typically based upon responses to one question, but the same pattern is visible in longitudinal studies. It's seen in both sexes, though men tend to be happier than women (although women smile more), and researchers have even claimed to have detected it in great apes.

A UK study that followed more than 9,000 people in their sixties for eight years found that people in the bottom quartile for happiness had a death rate of 29%. That rate fell to just 9% for those in the most contented quartile. Fittingly, some of this stark difference can be attributed to physical health.[26]

What causes happiness? The two main theories are economics and the effect of work on our well-being and psychology. We start off in life with high hopes, which we gradually realise are unlikely to be fulfilled; then middle age brings a new sense of realism, a determination to enjoy life as it is and thus an increase in happiness. I feel like mature runners simply bring more joy to running. We're no longer in it for the PBs, perhaps, and feel more motivated by the process or act of running itself. We also have far more knowledge about ourselves, our body and all its quirks. We've been here and done it before.

In summary

Ageing is terrifying. However we're led to believe that age-based physiological decline is inevitable, that we should just accept our fate and give in. But ageing is only half – or perhaps even less – down to our bodies and our cells. The other half comes from our lifestyles and the choices we make each day, about whether to drink alcohol, what time to go to bed, how much time we spend sitting down, whether to get our daps on and go for a run ...

We can turn back the clock. Long-term runners already experience many of the associated health benefits, including increased resistance to all the worst diseases, improved longevity and reversed ageing. If senescence can be accelerated – and the societal aggressive pursuit of comfort has done that – then it can also be slowed, have brakes applied to it and even be put into reverse gear.

The simple but profound act of running helps bone health and cardiovascular health, makes us more disease-resistant, increases longevity and healthspan, makes living right now better, and helps us mentally and intellectually. We don't actually decline all that fast; there are so many ageless aces to feel inspired by and age does have significant advantages.

We want to avoid injury or training breaks as a high priority to retain consistency that isn't just for performance but for age-resistant health, too. However, if we want to be the best athlete we can as we age, it's not quite as simple as 'keep calm and carry on'. We need to be a bit smarter than that ...

'You get older, but you mustn't treat yourself as old.'

JO PAVEY

Jo, fifty-two, became the oldest female European champion in history when she won the 10,000 metres gold at the 2014 European Championships aged forty, ten months after giving birth to her second child. Specialising in 5,000 metres and 10,000 metres, the World and Commonwealth medallist also ran in the 2016 Olympics one month before turning forty-three. Known for her signature, long compression socks which she felt helped her calves, she's the only British track athlete to have competed in five Olympic Games. Jo is also a physiotherapist, a *Runner's World* columnist and an ambassador for Running at 40 Plus.

Ageing for me was in two parts. As I got older, I was pleasantly surprised that I could keep going and was very fortunate to go to a fifth Olympics when I was almost forty-three. I got a lot of banter after I won the Europeans at forty. I got a new surname, 'Pavey forty', and my teammates called me Granny. At the Rio Olympics, my two teammates were twenty years younger than me and everyone else my age was in team management.

To still be competitive in my forties, I had to adapt my training. I would prioritise the most important sessions for my events. On the track, I knew what sessions worked for me and what times I needed to be hitting, for kilometre reps, for 400 metres. I also prioritised listening to my body, being more flexible, strength and conditioning, and doing a bit less volume, so I could maximise my recovery for the next key workout.

I was always trying to find a way. If I got a niggle, I would think, *What can I do, what alternative training?* I'm still training, I'm on a schedule, but I need a different mode of training. My favourite was aqua running, where I could train the hardest.

I kept going for a lot of years. It was partly the mental side, enjoying it, enjoying setting myself goals, enjoying working towards the next thing. Always the next thing, to aim for something new, to try different events. Plus not seeing stopping as an option. Not getting annoyed about being injured, just thinking how to find a way around it, rather than taking lay-offs.

Experience is definitely an advantage. You have more knowledge of your sport and, even more importantly, knowledge of what works for you. It's about learning what training mix works; knowing where strength and conditioning might fit, or where the mileage fits, or how much recovery you need after your long run to still be able to do a decent track session, the whole structure of your training week or cycle. As I got older, I made the cycle longer, so I could get all the key units in, extend the week a bit more, to eight or ten days.

It becomes easier to know what you need to do to get your best performances. I learned how to taper better, which is a massive thing for runners and really hard to get right. It's quite individual. And you learn more about what fuel you need and what your suitable race weight is

– you must be a healthy weight, where you're not getting run-down or injured. Knowing what a good pre-race meal is is important, too.

I got better at preparing for events mentally. At my first world championships I felt physically sick, and as a teenager I used to be sick sometimes. Later, I was still nervous, but in a way where I could control my nerves, use it to my advantage, channel that energy positively. As you get older, you've been in so many races, you know tactically how to get the best out of yourself.

When you're younger, you have a potentially faster body, but you're doing a lot of things wrong. You're overtrained for races, you aren't tapering enough, you eat something suboptimal, or you don't have much tactical awareness. At the start of my career I did a lot of hard sessions, but I wasn't always recovered for them. You learn how to recover well, too.

During my time on the British team, a lot of athletes came and went. I was always having different teammates. Generally, people would come along and have one or two good years and, unfortunately, they'd be lost to injury. I managed to keep myself healthy. I always had a regular menstrual cycle, whereas some women were not taking on enough energy to sustain themselves. That was a big thing. You need to look after your health. You need to take on enough energy.

It was fun seeing how far I could take it. I didn't really notice age hugely till I was about forty-six. I won the Vitality 10K in 2017 aged forty-three, but at about forty-five or forty-six I first noticed I was getting more nervous before some of my workouts, especially repeat 400 metres. I used to find I could do them in a good time, regardless of fitness. But it got to the point where that didn't happen any more. Even if I trained quite hard and felt I was doing them just as quick, the watch was saying no. That was a key session and I wasn't able to take it in my stride any more – literally. It just got harder to hit the targets. It was a realisation during track sessions over a couple of years, it felt unrealistic to run times that were good enough.

It was around the time of the pandemic that I lost the momentum of my competitive career. I was forty-six or forty-seven and I'm not saying I would have made the British team for the Tokyo Olympics, but I was trying to. I trained extremely hard all winter, but when the lockdown hit Devon I couldn't get to a track. You had to be a professional sportsperson, like at Loughborough or Birmingham, to have access. It's really hilly on the roads here – I could only find 27 seconds of flat. I couldn't really do the quality work. I was home-schooling both our kids and I didn't have access to a track for thirteen months. By the time the pandemic was over, I was so much older and then everything else started coming into play, a lot of family reasons, I was busy too, involved in running in different ways. I was forty-seven and I'd lost that momentum. I've just kind of accepted it.

Perimenopause makes your body more unpredictable. I've had sweats, feeling a lot more tiredness and much worse sleep. As I've got older, I need to do strength and conditioning, because it works against age-related declines in muscle mass, one of the reasons you lose your speed. Diet as you get older as well; you need to think about protecting bones and muscles, and think about recovery a lot more.

You get older, but you also mustn't treat yourself as old. You do need to be careful not to get injured, but that's true at any age. If you stop doing the speed work, you get slower. At the start of my career, I used to take long breaks at the end of a season, then come back and get injured from being deconditioned. I would also be surprised how hard it was to even do one lap at the pace I wanted to. Because I'd stopped doing the work. If you stop, you get slower anyway. So it's about not treating yourself as old. Instead, think, *Right, what have I got to do?*

I'm fifty-two now. I still love running, but I can't target PBs or compete for the British team. I accept that and I'm happy with that. Nowadays it's just loving getting out for a run, being part of running communities, keeping involved in sport in different ways. My husband's coaching a lot of athletes and I enjoy helping mentor them; I'm involved with Running at 40 Plus, getting people running above the age of forty; I really love working for *Runner's World*, writing a column about getting older as a runner. And I still have aspirations to achieve goals.

But as you get older, you really take on board how much running does for you. I appreciate more than ever the benefits of physical health and mental health and just enjoy getting out for a run. The social side of it, the camaraderie, the mental well-being of running in nature, and you appreciate more than ever how you love running. I'm still getting out every day and I want to keep going, just reaping the benefits it gives.

PART THREE: THE UGLY

'We don't stop running because we get old.
We get old because we stop running.'
ANONYMOUS

That's a great mantra for us masters runners. We should remind ourselves of it every day. We know lifestyle contributes to at least half, maybe much more, of our ageing process and we can push back, slow, pause and reverse it to an extent. Yes, ageing is inevitable. But *how we age* is a choice.

As the previous two sections showed, the bad news is that as we get older almost everything gets worse physiologically. The good news is that running is about the best thing we can do to push back against senescence, and continuing to strive for athletic excellence is proven to add years to our life. The ugly news is that us older dogs need to learn new tricks. We need to put the work in. Not necessarily more miles – in fact, probably fewer. We need to put in hard and fast miles. You know, the ones that make you gurn (puking is optional). And, #sorrynotsorry, but we need to get to the gym and/or invest in some kettlebells. We also need to rethink sleep, diet and our mindset. It may be uncomfortable at times. But it will all be worth it.

Before we get to all that, though, many runners will have to contend with the curveball of the ironically named menopause ...

MASTERING MENOPAUSE BY RENEE MCGREGOR

One of the things I find so fascinating about the human body is that it never stops evolving; whether we are talking about mental or physical health, humans generally don't stand still. Some of this we influence via our lifestyle choices, such as diet and exercise, but some of this is biological, like ageing.

No matter what we do, there are aspects of ageing we can't change or stop. One such situation is women's decline in their reproductive health as they go through perimenopause and menopause. This is a biological process that every woman is going to encounter. The exact date and how they experience it is very much an individual process, which not only makes it hard to identify at times but can also leave some women feeling confused as to why their symptoms are so different from their peers'.

Indeed, when we talk about this time of life, no one size fits all, but understanding how it can impact you, learning how your body works and learning how to respond will support your running as you enter perimenopause and get to the other side of menopause.

Perimenopause and menopause are often used interchangeably and yet they are different.

Perimenopause, or menopause transition, begins several years prior to menopause. It usually starts in a woman's forties but can start earlier and can last anything from a few months to ten years. Recently, the British Menopause Society reported that perimenopausal symptoms can start anywhere from five to seven years prior to actually going through menopause. The symptoms are associated with declining and fluctuating levels of the hormones oestrogen and progesterone.

Perimenopause stops at **menopause**, when the ovaries no longer produce any eggs and oestrogen and progesterone levels are low. The average age is fifty-one. This means most women will experience symptoms in their early forties but may not even be aware of this, especially as early symptoms are not always recognisable. It's also important to highlight that women who go through an early menopause may start showing signs of perimenopause in their mid- to late thirties.

The importance of oestrogen and progesterone

While there is a lot of negative press about hormones and menstruation, having a period is actually a good sign and a real barometer of health. It's basically saying that conditions are optimal for a pregnancy to occur. However, a period is more than just a reproductive portal. Contrary to what you may have read, **oestrogen** has a diverse role within the body. While it is a reproductive hormone, its benefits for women and their health are widespread, including cognitive function, balance, proprioception, heart health, immune health and mood. This is why as levels start to decline we can experience such a mixed range of symptoms.

Hormones are chemical messengers made by specialised cells within endocrine glands, responsible for the correct function of the body. We have a long list of hormones all working together, helping to monitor the body based on a series of feedback loops. They all have critical roles to play, from maintaining metabolic function to ensuring progression and adaptation from our training, optimising bone health, appetite control and sleep regulation.

Therefore, regulating and maintaining our hormonal health, for both males and females, is central to both our health and performance, and understanding how to harness the benefits of these amazing chemical messengers allows us to meet our potential.

Oestrogen is produced by both males and females. Its key role is in the regulation and maintenance of a healthy reproductive system. However, due to the higher levels in women, its influence goes further, with positive effects on skin, connective tissue, heart, bone and brain health. Thus as levels decline, we may start to see specific changes to these areas. In fact, low mood and higher anxiety are two of the most overlooked early signs of perimenopause.

Progesterone, another key reproductive hormone, plays a role in regulating the menstrual cycle, supporting pregnancy, and influencing mood, sleep and other bodily functions. Its decline during perimenopause can lead to irregular periods, mood swings and sleep disturbances.

Signs and symptoms

Until recently, menopause was rarely spoken about and the term perimenopause wasn't even in our medical vocabulary. The increased awareness and discussion is so important, but some people are still quite confused as to what this phase of life means. Most women I speak to assume they can't be going through the perimenopause because they are still having regular periods, yet because symptoms can start five to seven years ahead of actually going through menopause, many women continue to have a regular menstrual cycle, and this is one of the last aspects to disappear.

Loss of menstruation should never be ignored, but it should also not be immediately assumed that if it's lost during a woman's forties she is perimenopausal. Similarly, a medic should not wait for this sign before providing care for a woman with perimenopausal symptoms.

Perimenopause is a time when hormones are constantly fluctuating, and this is why every woman's experience will be so individual. Diagnosis and identification is tricky as there are no real blood tests and, to date, medical providers are advised to make a diagnosis through clinical questioning and the symptoms being experienced.

There are in the region of 200 potential symptoms which would indicate a woman might be going through perimenopause, but we only tend to hear about the most common, such as hot flushes, fatigue, brain fog and joint pain. Other lesser-known symptoms include digestive changes, low mood, changes to sport performance, dry eyes, dry skin, restless legs, an increase in urinary tract infections and heightened anxiety.

While symptoms will vary from woman to woman, some of the most commonly reported include:

- lower sex drive
- hot flushes
- worsening premenstrual symptoms
- fatigue
- irregular periods
- vaginal dryness and discomfort during sex
- urinary leakage when coughing or sneezing
- mood swings
- heightened anxiety and sense of dissociation
- low mood
- sleep disturbances
- joint pain
- poor memory
- low iron levels
- palpitations.

While this list looks daunting, it is important to stress that there is also no way of predicting which symptoms you may experience, their intensity or when during your perimenopausal years they might occur. Mood and anxiety-related symptoms may show up earlier in the journey and be overlooked as a stressful time, rather than recognising they could be the start of perimenopause. Similarly, some women will sail through with no symptoms whatsoever except in the last few months before they complete menopause, while others may end up having several of the symptoms consistently or at least cyclically throughout their journey.

However, it's not all doom and gloom. While perimenopause and menopause are poorly researched areas of female health, in recent years they have started to get some airtime and awareness, especially as improved nutrition, lifestyle and medicine means that so many of us in the Western world live longer and want to maintain a certain quality of life for as long as possible. Advances in our understanding of how this stage of life impacts women, and improvement in medicines, mean there are many approaches available that can alleviate symptoms. No one needs to suffer during this stage of life. My advice is to make sure you get the help you need – and that doesn't always mean HRT.

Bone health

While it is a concern for most women, runners who are going through the perimenopause are most likely aware of and concerned about how this stage of life has a negative impact on bone health. As we age, bone health declines in both men and women, but there is an increased drop-off in women due to the decline in production of oestrogen.

Key facts:

- Hip fracture in women is more common than breast, uterine and ovarian cancer combined.
- One in two women (and one in five men) will get osteoporosis.
- There is a 25% drop in bone density in the ten years around perimenopause.

Bone health is one of those things we seem to take for granted. While 90% of adult bone mass is in place by the end of adolescence, continuing to look after our bones into adulthood is still really important.

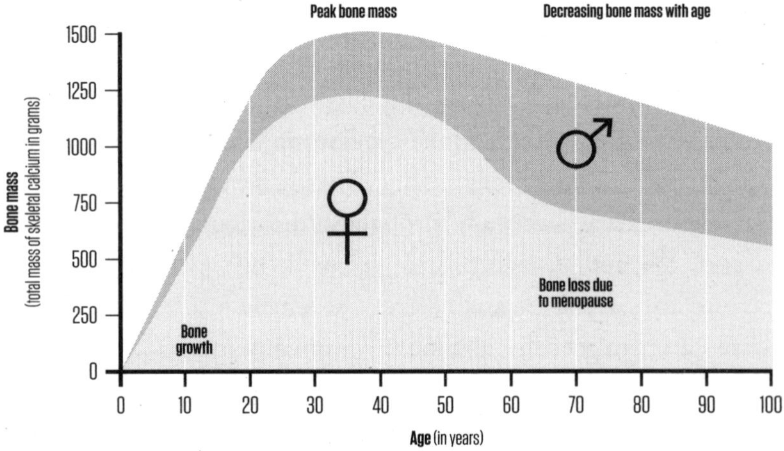

Graph depicting the relation between bone mass and age in males and females. © *Anatomy and Physiology* (2022), OpenStax, Creative Commons Attribution 4.0 International (CC BY)

Bone density naturally starts to decline from our late twenties. While genetics do have a part to play in our overall bone health and strength, the process of decline can be preserved or accelerated by a number of nutritional, lifestyle and environmental factors.

The key influencers in maintaining bone health are exercise, nutrition and hormones.

Nutrition plays a critical role in bone health, with key nutrients being calcium, phosphorus, magnesium, and vitamins D, C and K. While it is essential to include these nutrients in appropriate quantities, it is important to be aware that if the energy intake is insufficient to meet the demands of the body, these nutrients in isolation can do little for our bone health.

Oestrogen plays a huge part in maintaining optimal bone health. Adequate levels of these hormones are maintained through ensuring good intakes of energy, especially carbohydrate. This is why the incidence of osteoporosis increases so significantly in postmenopausal women and is one of the main reasons we encourage women of a certain age to *consider* taking hormone replacement therapy.

While we can't negate the effects of declining oestrogen levels, staying physically active and doing weight-bearing exercise has been shown to have a positive impact on bone health. In fact, as we get older, studies suggest there may be more benefit for women in reducing run volume and increasing strength and resistance training. The mechanical loading of the skeleton is essential for the maintenance of normal bone mass and architecture. Activities that involve plyometric and change-of-direction movements, as well as isometric exercises that place force on the bone, are particularly useful and should be introduced during the perimenopause, especially if they have not previously featured (see page 98 for more).

To ensure that you are looking after your bones:

- Exercise regularly. While running is a great weight-bearing sport, it only supports unidirectional movement. Bones really like a variety of movements to ensure they get the stimulus they need to become strong and supportive. This means adding in multidirectional movement, plyometrics and also heavy load. Thus it is beneficial to also include resistance training, band work, skipping or team sports such as hockey, netball or football.

- Take a vitamin D supplement, especially if your levels are below the recommended values for health. For runners, the normal acceptable parameters are too low and you should aim for a value of at least 75 nanograms per litre.
- Ensure you are getting sufficient calcium intake. Perimenopausal women should aim for 1,000 milligrams of calcium a day, with menopausal women increasing this to 1,200 milligrams. Consuming at least three to four servings of dairy/soya a day can support this, where one serving is the equivalent to:
  - a 300-millilitre glass of milk, either cow's or soya
  - a matchbox-sized portion of cheese
  - a (150-gram) pot of yoghurt, either cow's or soya
  - 100 grams of cottage cheese
  - a 100-gram serving of tofu.
- Include plenty of fruits and vegetables; potato skins, berries and oranges are high in vitamin C, while dark green leafy vegetables are high in vitamin K.

What about energy availability?

Even if we are putting in the right building blocks of nutrition, if our overall energy intake – and specifically carbohydrate intake – is not sufficient, then no amount of supplementing is going to support optimal bone health. Bone activity is highest in the immediate phase post-run, so while it's really important to fuel each run with sufficient carbohydrate, it's equally important to ensure that we replenish the tank with a good intake of carbohydrate and protein, ideally within 30 minutes of our run. If this can't be our next meal, chocolate milk or soya milk can be really good choices as they deliver hydration, carbohydrate, protein and calcium all in one hit.

One key point, though: not all plant-based drinks are equal. Soya is by far the best choice if we want to hit our calcium and protein intake.

Many women going through perimenopause struggle with changes to their body composition. I want to stress here that it's completely normal for the female body to change in shape and composition as hormonal levels decline. Cue current misconceptions and Western societal beliefs, and many women at this stage decide that the only way to combat this change is through restrictive diets and, in particular, removing carbohydrates.

In fact, the latest research shows women should do the complete opposite: declining oestrogen levels mean that the female body is no longer efficient at fat oxidation, which tends to spare our use of carbohydrates. Thus carbohydrate intake, especially in women who remain physically active, is critical not just for performance but also for counteracting the fatigue often associated with this phase of life. While intermittent fasting and keto diets are widely promoted by celebrities and popular media, these approaches can actually have a worsening impact on quality of life, health and definitely physical performance.

There is a direct link between carbohydrate availability and thyroid function. A recent study by Danish researcher Anna Melin confirmed that carbohydrate availability plays a key role in hormonal regulation and menstrual health, particularly in women who are physically active. In fact, when carbohydrate intake is reduced drastically in females of any age, there is a reduction in the production of thyroid hormones T3 and T4, resulting in a down-regulation of metabolism, impacting body composition and energy levels further. Additional research suggests that when T4 is particularly low, this stops the production of one of our key performance hormones, IGF-1.

The gut microbiome

Another area that often gets overlooked during perimenopause is the gut microbiome. While this is still a relatively new area of nutrition, numerous studies have demonstrated that there is no denying a link between the status of our gut microbiome and both our mental and physical health.

The gut microbiome includes a different type of bacteria that reside in our gut. Collectively, these have a number of functions, including synthesising some vitamins, short-chain fatty acids and even neurotransmitters, which are all necessary for optimal health.

The more enriched microbial diversity an individual has, the more likely they are to benefit from the positive associations with health. These include a strong immune system and improved mental health, and more recently there seem to be links with improvements to sports performance.

As women go through the perimenopause, hormonal changes can result in gut dysbiosis, a change to the microbial diversity which can impact digestion and also health.

While research around the microbiome and women's health is emerging, it does appear to confirm that the production of oestrogen and the gut biome are a bidirectional process – that is, oestrogen influences the gut biome, but equally the gut biome impacts the production of oestrogen.

During perimenopause and then menopause, the reduction in oestrogen appears to have a direct impact on the production of certain bacteria in the gut microbiome. This can lead to further dysbiosis during this period of life and appears to be related to some of the symptoms most commonly associated with menopause, such as hot flushes and night sweats. Practically, in my own work, I have also witnessed that in this group of women, levels of iron – particularly the stores, ferritin and B12 – appear to drop, further impacting fatigue and general feelings of well-being. While there don't appear to be any studies looking at this specifically, it would make sense that dysbiosis would interfere with the absorption of these nutrients. Additionally, production of intrinsic factor, which is a glycoprotein that binds with B12 and helps absorption, reduces with age and can also be significantly impacted by changes in digestion and the gut microbiome. I would highly recommend that women in this population group regularly check levels of both these nutrients to ensure they are not deficient. However, more research is needed to confirm this.

Similarly, to date, there doesn't appear to be any research on how the use of HRT may influence or impact the gut microbiome. With all this in mind, it's worth considering making appropriate nutritional choices that can support gut health, especially if there is a chance it can not only support running performance but also reduce the risk of certain perimenopausal symptoms.

'I have a mantra: I can only do what I can do today.'

SUSIE CHAN

Susie, fifty, is an endurance runner, Peloton instructor and author of the award-winning *Trails and Tribulations*. She's completed numerous 100-mile races, including the Marathon des Sables in the Sahara Desert four times and the notorious 135-mile Badwater ultramarathon. She also broke the world record for the furthest distance run on a treadmill in 12 hours. Susie has used her large social media following to discuss her journey through menopause.

I collapsed at the end of the Chicago Marathon. I was pursuing the World Marathon Majors and I had this dreadful cough. It just wouldn't go for about five months, and it was absolutely diabolical at Chicago. But I wanted my Six Star medal! I was coughing my way around and I was like, 'Whatever happens, don't let them take me off the course.' I got the Six Star and just collapsed.

I had an X-ray and they found an enormous lump in my neck, absolutely huge. I had to have it taken out. It was a strange way to find out I had cancer. I missed one ultramarathon and I remember being very upset about that.

I dealt with it by running. I did a half-marathon two weeks later, which I definitely shouldn't have done. I did Marathon des Sables about five weeks later, then Keys 100 in Florida a month later, and I did a 24-hour track race that year, too. I was probably proving to myself that I could still do all the things I wanted to do. It was a shock. Because you're running around doing these extraordinary races and you think you're bulletproof, invincible. But your own body is conspiring against you. That was a bit of a moment.

Menopause has been miserable. Overall it's been net grim. I think because I run, the experience is more exacerbated. If I didn't run, I'd probably only really feel how hard it was when I'd push myself doing some kind of fitness. So if I didn't like to ultra-run for a living, it would probably be manageable, you know. But when I push myself, it's really hard.

Running exposes your weaknesses very, very easily. If you run a long way, you're going to find out exactly where you're weak, particularly with my body going through the changes it's going through now. I'm being hyper aware of what I can no longer do and what is more challenging now. At first, I felt really tired and really sluggish. Sometimes when I'm having a tough week, it's like somebody has sucked all the fitness out of my body. The other week, I couldn't string three miles together. I just couldn't do it. I was absolutely fucked. The major symptom I've had, which has been really annoying, is my joints hurt. My hands will be hurting. My shoulders will be aching. I just wake up feeling knackered; I'll get cramps, like menstrual cramps; I get dizzy sometimes. Sometimes it's one or two of those, sometimes it's all of them.

It's unpredictable and it's very hard to know how I'm going to feel on any given day. It's knocked my confidence. I feel a lot less confident about race performances. Will I even finish? Will it be a dreadful day, or will it be an okay day? So that's hard to manage sometimes. As positive as I am, some days are like, 'For fuck sake, why am I doing this again? Why don't I just go and do something else?'

Maybe it's the ultrarunner in me, but I refuse to just resign myself to it and stop running. I love running. I love the people I run with, I love the community, I love my job. So I won't stop. I'll just do what I can do on the day. And if it does mean I'm a lot slower, so be it. That just happens to be how I am. I have a philosophy for it, a mantra: I can only do what I can do on that day.

Post-cancer I've never been able to run like I could before. The pursuit of enjoyment, for me, is a lot less about my minute miles and much more about experiences now. I chose to go to more races with my friends. My fondest running memories aren't like, 'Oh, I hit every split at the Berlin Marathon!' Instead, I think about being with amazing people in a desert, or an amazing weekend away with my friends running a marathon. After cancer, I decided to pursue a route which was more fun. It's very liberating when you don't give a shit about your times any more.

But I did go through a spell where I found the adjustment mentally very, very tough. Because I couldn't run a 6:50 mile any more and I was sort of chasing it and chasing it. You're on Strava, people are watching your runs, you're posting about your race times, being in this social media age we live in, and I suddenly couldn't run like I used to. You get anxious and you're just dreading running.

Then I went through a whole process of just accepting it. You can't keep getting faster. You can't keep hitting marathons at the same pace. And I got over the ego attached to that, which was good, because I got that out of the way in my early forties.

I don't put any pressure on myself with time goals any more. I did a 50K race recently and I walked a lot because the weather was awful, and in my head it was like, *Oh God, not this again.* But I just kept moving forward. And of course, when I finished, I was delighted. I was really glad I did it. I was really glad I didn't just walk to my car, give up and drive home. I still achieved what I wanted to achieve that day, which was a race finish, as best I could do it. So it is a lot about reframing and just being kind to yourself in those moments.

The experience of sharing my menopause experience publicly has been very positive. It's just nice to know you're not alone, that there's hundreds of other women in the same boat. Whenever I speak about it, I get women being like, 'Oh, thank goodness you're speaking about it. It's been really nice to hear somebody else saying they're having a harder day today – and that that's okay.' Fifty per cent of the population will have this and it's very under-researched and under-communicated.

I haven't made it my entire personality yet, but it's something I'm leaning into. I can't change what's happening, but I can create my own narrative of how I'm dealing with it. It's happening. So I either choose to accept it and look for the bits which are rewarding and positive, or I could let it take over my life and just be miserable about it. And I'm absolutely refusing to do that.

The perimenopausal runner

If we think research is limited in female athletes, try finding research in perimenopausal and postmenopausal athletes. Until recently, most female athletes would retire from their sporting careers in their mid- to late thirties. While this may still be the case in several sports and at an elite level, more and more women are continuing to compete well into their forties, fifties and sixties. Age-group triathlon, masters running events and the rise of ultra-endurance events, where being an older female may even be an advantage, all encourage participation.

To date, there are no studies that look specifically at athletic performance in this population group, but there is good evidence to back up regular exercise as a way to mitigate some of the more unpleasant aspects of going through the perimenopause.

The most common symptoms most women report and worry about include:

- fatigue
- less adaptation from training load
- changes to body composition.

It's important to highlight that many factors may contribute to these symptoms. Lower levels of both oestrogen and progesterone are likely to result in poor sleep. Sleep is one of the most underrated influencers of optimal recovery, from activity and life itself. Appropriate sleep has a direct correlation with our psychological and physical health. Thus poor sleep will contribute to inadequate recovery from exercise performance, which in turn may make physical activity feel a lot harder. Decrease in activity due to fatigue, and a lower motivation to train due to poor recovery, has implications for our body composition, which often goes hand in hand with perimenopause.

Additionally, it has been well documented that muscle mass and strength declines through ageing, and in particular bone health declines more rapidly in women. In general, muscle mass and strength peaks between the ages of twenty and thirty, and begins to decline from forty to fifty, with an acceleration in decline in the over-seventies.

One key finding from the research across all masters age groups is that any decline in muscle mass is directly linked with physical activity, with inactive and sedentary peers experiencing a more rapid decline.

Resistance training seems to be pivotal in maintaining mass in this population. The inclusion of two or three sessions a week, potentially even replacing one or two runs a week, can reap huge benefits and also help manage overall fatigue and stress on the body, and mitigate some of the changes to body composition. Remember that maintaining muscle mass also means maintaining metabolism.

Training around perimenopause and menopause

As previously indicated, scientific evidence demonstrates that being active actually supports this stage of life. Regular activity can help with mood and body composition, can improve the management of most symptoms (with the exception of hot flushes), and also reduces the risk of heart disease, which rises as a direct response to lower oestrogen levels. For women who have always been sedentary, this may be the perfect time to start getting active.

Specifically, it has been suggested that women should include 2 hours and 30 minutes of aerobic/endurance-based exercise a week, two strength/resistance training sessions a week, and one breath-based exercise such as yoga or t'ai chi to minimise stress and support overall well-being.

However, care needs to be taken in women who have been shown to have low bone density and osteoporosis, especially if they are new to resistance training. Additionally, this particular group may need to avoid high-impact, high-intensity training. Working with a qualified coach who can advise on appropriate training load across both aerobic and resistance training is advised.

But what if you are someone who has been competitive or used to a high training load and is noticing a decline in performance or an inability to maintain previous levels?

HRV

HRV (heart rate variability) measures the tiny variations in the time intervals between consecutive heartbeats, indicating how well our autonomic nervous system is balancing the 'fight or flight' (sympathetic) and 'rest and digest' (parasympathetic) systems. Higher HRV generally signifies a resilient body that can adapt to stress, while lower HRV can indicate stress, illness or overtraining. It's available on many GPS sports watches and apps now and is a personalised measure best compared with our own baseline trends rather than with others.

A recent study has shown correlation between a low HRV and more intense menopausal symptoms. Moreover, it highlights how the process of perimenopause – the constant fluctuations and the unpredictable nature of symptoms – generates stress within the body. Many women are unaware of this and often question why their HRV takes a sudden drop, even when their overall training and life load appears normal.

It's important to remember that the human body doesn't differentiate stress from physical, biological, lifestyle or psychological factors. Stress is stress and, while we need some stress, when our central nervous system becomes overloaded, it starts to have a negative impact on our body. The stress associated with going through perimenopause may not always be easy to pick up, and many women, especially those of us who are used to being physically active, find it confusing as to why their body is suddenly no longer feeling able.

This is why understanding and monitoring HRV is a useful tool for women to use, to help them to respond to their body and manage training load. What I will emphasise is that HRV is a gauge, and you most definitely don't want to live your life by it. Learning to listen and respond to your body is key, but monitoring HRV can provide you with some reassurance and accountability.

HRT

HRT (hormone replacement therapy) is an effective treatment for improving menopausal symptoms and protecting bone health in many women. However, while there are often significant health benefits, it is a personal choice, with many women being wary, some women being unable to take it due to medical unsuitability and some women finding that it just doesn't improve their symptoms. Like the perimenopausal journey itself, the use of HRT will vary from individual to individual with regard to type, dose and even how long a person stays on it.

Previously, there was a lot of negative press associated with HRT. This was mainly based on the outcome of the 2002 Women's Health Initiative Study, which has since been criticised for providing misinformation. It looked at outcomes in women over sixty who were given a type of HRT that is no longer in common use, and concluded that in this group there was a higher incidence of breast cancer as a direct result of taking the HRT. However, it is also well documented that our risk of getting breast cancer increases over the age of sixty.

Similarly, women who have previously had breast cancer and have had to go through a medically induced menopause should be aware of the use of HRT. It is always best to discuss each case with the breast and oncology team, alongside a menopause specialist GP where possible.

HRT consists of replacing the hormones that have declined through menopause, namely oestrogen and progesterone. Oestrogen is most commonly used transdermally (through the skin as a patch, gel or spray), as this is the lowest risk approach. Women who still have their uterus (so they have not had a hysterectomy) also need a form of progesterone to protect the uterine lining. This may be in the form of tablets, the Mirena coil or even a progesterone-only pill. The latter two options also provide ongoing contraceptive protection, which is advised in women until the age of fifty-five unless menopause has been confirmed at an earlier age.

There are many variations of HRT available. It is not a one-size-fits-all treatment and it may take a few months to work out what dose is best for you.

It's important to highlight that HRT is ideally used to manage and improve perimenopausal symptoms. This means it may well improve symptoms associated with a reduction in performance, such as fatigue. Indeed, many women who take HRT report benefits, but it is by no means performance-enhancing. That said, some women may be prescribed testosterone as part of their HRT routine. Testosterone is a banned substance in sport and so women who want to remain competitive may have to avoid the use of this hormone.

One final point: HRT is not for everybody and no woman should feel forced into this decision. Lifestyle behaviours around nutrition and activity, as we have discussed above, can all support this period of time. Equally, no one also needs to suffer or be fearful. Remember that HRT is something you can always experiment with until you find the right option, or decide that it is not for you.

Perimenopause and mental health

While this chapter has mainly focused on the physical symptoms of perimenopause, it feels important to also include some of the issues that can occur with our mental health. Remember, our mind and body are not separate entities and it can be important to look at our whole self.

Brain health is an area that needs more investigation, especially when it comes to the perimenopause and menopause. We know that altering hormonal levels lead to many of the symptoms associated with this period of life. Brain fog and changes to our cognition are well documented, but evidence is emerging that there may also be structural and neurotransmitter production changes that leave us feeling a bit off kilter.

Perimenopause often coincides with big life changes, such as children leaving the family home, caring for ageing parents and elevated risk to personal health. The combination of these factors, including just dealing with the fluctuating hormonal levels, can often leave a woman feeling out of sorts and messy, perhaps with a sense of falling short or even being unworthy. Humans are hardwired to avoid threat and many of us will look for ways to avoid some of these uncomfortable emotions and feelings that are bubbling away under the surface.

Eating disorders and exercise dependency are two such methods of coping that provide distraction, a false sense of security and a method of avoiding feeling. Fixation on how to eat and what to eat can initially feel like an escape, but as with all false refuges, the relief is temporary. An eating disorder can soon spiral and result in biological consequences that are harmful to health. Similarly, using exercise as a way of avoidance may seem harmless, but if it becomes something you can't live without, it can lead to negative consequences to health.

Individually or combined, these two particular 'coping mechanisms' can also be the precursor to REDs (relative energy deficiency in sport). This is when there is insufficient energy in the body relative to the work being asked of it, where work is all movement and biological function. The symptoms of REDs can also be very similar to perimenopause, and can run in parallel to it, adding complexity to the picture.

Women who have previously suffered with mental illness such as eating disorders or depression earlier in their life are probably the most susceptible, especially if they didn't fully understand the true purpose of their dysfunctional behaviour.

As with all mental illness, seeking help from a team of qualified practitioners is advised and recommended.

In summary

It is clear that while going through perimenopause and menopause is not a new phenomenon, it is only really in the last three to five years that the spotlight has been placed on this topic, in an attempt to raise awareness and improve quality of life during this final third of a woman's lifespan.

There is still a lot we do not know, but what is clear is that it's a huge time of transition, both physically and emotionally. I often describe it as puberty in reverse, where every day feels like a new experience and it can be hard to predict how we might feel or what we are able to do. However, the more we can inform and empower women to become aware of their bodies and encourage less comparison to our peers, the easier this period becomes to navigate. While this is an individual journey, it is good to know there are many more options available than once thought. Support is available.

The final words I want to leave with you are **learn to listen**. Appreciate that this is a time of change, and one that can leave you feeling vulnerable at times. That is definitely not a weakness but indeed a strength. By listening in, you can learn to respond in a way that is nurturing, compassionate and more respectful towards your body and mind.

Thanks to Dr Cath Munro for her help in checking the HRT section of this chapter.

'Age can definitely be an advantage, in racing and in training.'

HOLLY STABLES

Holly (who competed as Holly Rush until 2021), forty-eight, is an international road marathon runner turned ultra-trail runner. She represented Great Britain at the European Athletics Championships (team silver medallists) and Commonwealth Games (placing eighth) in 2010. She won the Pisa and Edinburgh marathons, before graduating to ultra distance and taking first place at Ultravasan and seventh place at the historic Comrades Marathon, while also representing GB at the World Mountain Championships (winning team silver and bronze). Also a running coach, Holly has won numerous trail-ultramarathons, including placing second overall at the Speed Project Solo, a 340-mile, unsanctioned race across the desert from Los Angeles to Las Vegas, aged forty-seven.

You can take getting old in different ways: a change in the way you look physically, or a change in how you're performing. I was like a lot of female marathon runners, very aware of the way I looked on the start line. We'd be wearing a crop top and knickers, which when you think about it is pretty awful, because you're standing there in your underwear. I always felt very funny about that, felt like I was bigger, even though I'm sure that was massive body dysmorphia.

Since I moved towards ultras in 2013, I've been much happier with how I look physically, how much more athletic and stronger I feel now than I ever did in my twenties and thirties. When I first started doing strength training, in my early forties, my bum had slipped down the back of my legs. Everything was slipping down, all going to be found in my socks. I think I look way better physically now and I feel so much better. Not my face. My face looks like a tea bag.

In terms of my performance, I was fed up with competitive marathon running and switched to ultras before I started to slow down. I fell out of love with training for marathons, because I saw no progression after a while. My relationship was very goal-driven, very stats-driven. I just found it all-consuming and I needed to break from it.

I came to terms with the fact I wasn't going to run under 2:40 ever again. I remind myself that I am a 2:37 marathon runner and no one can take that away from me. I'm proud of that and I'm proud that I went to all those international championships. When I have run marathons since, I'm around 5–10 minutes slower than my PB. I have come to terms with that. But I found it quite hard.

I haven't seen a big deterioration, probably because I've been so consistent the last seven years. From the age of about forty-six, maybe the last couple of years, I have seen more of a drop-off with speed. Back in the day, my 10-mile or half-marathon pace was around 5:35-minute mileing and marathon was 6-minute mileing, but now my race pace for 10K, half marathon and marathon is almost the same. I had some promising workouts at the beginning of this year, though, things in the 5-minute mile stuff, which was surprising.

I want to be competitive in ultras, like the South Downs Way 50K this year [where Holly placed second in a competitive field]. I was slightly miffed about being ranked sixth. I thought, *Sod that, I'm gonna give it some welly.* The girls went off quite hard and I watched them from behind, content with letting them go. I knew that pace was completely fine for me but if I pushed it any further I might pay for it later; whereas before I probably would have not been confident enough in my ability and tried to go with them. With age and experience, I'm just a little bit more like 'No, this is the right effort for me and I know later I should pick up places.'

Age can definitely be an advantage. I understand the effort I'm putting in better now, that experience of how your body feels in races. And I think it's about being confident. Even if I didn't think I could be competitive, I'm still going to work really hard, I'm going to be running for a time, or for myself. I'm not going to be running for a place and I'm okay with that. But in ultras, for now, I'm running to be competitive and place.

Next year I want to try Cocodona 250 [a 250-mile race in Arizona], because that would just be horrendous and I might be terrible at it. But I need to do something that's different and just see what happens. I will always prepare as well as I can and be in the best position possible when I line up. And if someone beats me and I'm giving it 100%, then they're better than me and I will congratulate them. That's fine.

My training has changed. I was doing high mileage, with doubles, averaging around 100 miles a week. I was doing two or three workouts a week and no strength training. It was just stupid. And I was running way faster on my easy runs, which makes me laugh. I've got books and books and books of all my training diaries, but I stopped filling them out when I started doing ultras. I've never written anything down since. It doesn't interest me. I purposely give myself two days easy after harder sessions now and I have one day off a week, which I never used to have. My strength training is almost as important as the running. I'm lifting four times a week. It's really, really important. I want to have muscle. For me, it really is consistency.

If I do a session and it's going really well, I might say, actually, I'm not going to do the last rep, I'm going to leave it there. I'm good. I don't need to do any more. Or, I'm supposed to do a 24-mile run today, but actually I'm gonna do 20 miles, because I feel fine with that; whereas back in the day, I would beat myself up about not doing that last rep or extra miles.

I listen to my body more. And I eat way more protein. After sessions, I eat more food. I was appalling at eating and now it's completely different. I prioritise protein and just eating more food. I have to, because I broke down all the time.

I have a routine and it's pretty sad, but I stick to it. I go to bed early, half nine. I don't really drink any more. I don't do any other fancy things. I don't have recovery boots, I don't roll, I don't have massage guns, I don't do yoga, I don't stretch. I don't do anything like that. I do see a physio fairly regularly.

I had perimenopausal symptoms from forty-six. I had general lethargy – I just wanted to fall asleep in a hedge – and achy knees, but not in an injured way. I started on HRT and it's really helped me. If you're over forty, you're probably perimenopausal. Why not replace those natural hormones and feel twenty-one again?!

The other thing that you can't buy is just being happy, because I was desperately unhappy for a long, long time. And that has so many implications for how your body reacts to things. So I think being okay with life and your situation is really important. As you get older, you just become a little bit more content and a little bit, like, realistic. And you're not searching so much, are you, for something better?

My mum power-lifts. She's eighty and she deadlifts over 70 kilograms. She's a garden designer and a few years ago she couldn't lift up her watering can, she was taking so many pain meds for her back. She's had two frozen shoulders and she was really down. She started deadlifting and bench pressing and before you knew it, she was coming into the gym with a can of Monster, lifting and having a protein bar on the way out.

She used to say, 'Oh, I can't do that, I'm too tired.' Now she drives back from the gym with a smile on her face; she's so energised and she spends all day gardening: she digs, prunes hedges, she's up a ladder. She's stronger than my stepdad. I think she's stronger than me.

THE NEED FOR SPEED

If we intend to rage against the dying of the light, then we need to continue training consistently as if our life depends on it – because it kind of does.

Training consistently isn't just about parkrun. It's critical for our health. Midlife is forty for women, thirty-seven for men. From a health perspective, starting to think about longevity isn't just for seventy-year-olds. Remember, traces of future life-ending problems can present in our twenties and will often come to fruition before we're sixty-five. Simply put, the less fit we are, the closer to death we are. Lifestyle diseases, the Four Horsemen, are already working on us, especially if we're not prioritising our fitness.

'We need to pivot our mindsets,' says Dr Vonda Wright, orthopaedic surgeon and author of *Unbreakable: A Women's Guide to Aging with Power*. 'There's a pervasive myth that aging is an inevitable decline from the vitality of youth down some slippery slope to frailty where we spend the last twenty years of our lives dying,' she says. 'There's so much we can do to pre-plan our future.'

Finnish researchers discovered that **the decade from thirty-six to forty-six has the biggest impact on our health later in life**. Wright calls it 'the critical decade'. Our body is at a crossroads where bad habits are catching up, but we can still reverse most of the damage. After forty-six, changes become much harder and less effective. By thirty-six, many of us are settled in careers and relationships, and have perhaps co-created some mini humans. Not everyone has been prioritising an optimal lifestyle, though. There often doesn't feel like there's time.

'But we are still young enough, with youthful vigour and youngish stem cells, to course-correct,' says Wright. 'This is the time to develop the habits of mobility, to develop the habits of lifting weights, to look at what you're eating; there's also perimenopause ... If you get those habits established, it will not be such a shock as it is for those who come to my office at sixty-five and say, "Oh my god, what do I do now?"'

That said, no age is too late, she adds. 'Your body will always respond to the positive stress you put on it.' But like the *Titanic* heading towards an iceberg, the earlier we can course-correct, the better the chance of missing a prematurely messy ending.

So, the number one rule for the mature athlete is this: don't stop. The number two rule is the need for speed. While consistent training is crucial, simply doing what we've always done won't give us optimal benefits and may even be speeding us towards slowing down. If you remember nothing else from this book, it's the mantra 'use it or lose it'.

There are athletic advantages, but let's first look at the huge health ones. Our VO2 max or maximum aerobic capacity isn't just a good indicator of our marathon or parkrun PB potential. It's an indicator of our lifespan, a biomarker for ageing and disease resistance. 'It's the single most important metric for someone's longevity,' says biomedical scientist and health educator Dr Rhonda Patrick.

As we age, our lung function, heart rate, blood volume, oestrogen and testosterone all decline and we consequently lose strength, power and speed. If we do nothing about that, our maximal aerobic capacity decreases and we allow ourselves to slow – to age prematurely. We need to fight back, by keeping our top speed as high as possible. Our aerobic capacity isn't like aerobic endurance, which takes years to optimise and in turn lingers for years. It's the classic use it or lose it. If we don't run fast, we won't be fast.

A declining VO2 max signals mitochondrial dysfunction, poor metabolic flexibility and increased mortality risk; while increasing our aerobic capacity means reduced risks of heart disease, diabetes, cancer and stroke. Increasing our VO2 max might just be the biggest long-term athletic and health intervention we can make. 'It is one of the more malleable characteristics of ageing,' says Frank W. Booth, a professor of physiology at the University of Missouri. 'You want to fight like hell to keep your

VO2 max from falling if you want to keep your healthspan.'

Running fast brings more bonuses. It increases testosterone by 30% and growth hormone by 20% in men, increases positive hormonal responses in women, engages those precious fast-twitch fibres, burns 40% more fat while preserving lean muscle, aids bone density, strengthens joints and tendons, improves reaction time, resets our nervous system, lowers cortisol and improves cognitive sharpness. It's about the best biological insurance policy we can take out. So we have several very good reasons to keep our VO2 max high, including lifespan, healthspan and Strava.

That's a lot of reasons to run fast. If we stay fast, we're better athletes, and we live longer and better. At a certain age, we may not be getting any quicker. But if we keep hitting the right buttons, we won't be getting slower for a while yet.

Let's get into the sporting reasons to run hard and fast sometimes. We know from studies based on identical twins that VO2 max is largely determined by genetics, doesn't move that much in well-trained athletes and will have dropped if we haven't been doing regular VO2 max workouts. One of the original VO2 max studies, back in the 1930s, analysed sixteen elite runners for twenty-five years.[1] They included 2-mile world-record holder Don Lash, who had a very high VO2 max of 81.4 millilitres per kilogram per minute. Most well-trained runners would expect to be above 40 for women and above 50 for men; sub-three-hour marathoners above 60 in their peak years – though don't trust your watch's estimate. Twenty-five years later, Lash had continued training but his intensity had dropped, which led to his VO2 max decreasing to 54.4, a decline of 27%, albeit only roughly 1% per year. The other fifteen runners had all stopped training in the meantime and their VO2 max scores had dropped by 43%, around 2% per year. In terms of aerobic capacity, they were no different to sedentary men their age. So, sadly, **being someone who used to run a fair bit but doesn't often now doesn't count for that much physiologically.**

A watershed study by Dr Michael Pollock analysed twenty-four masters athletes over twenty years. After ten years, the eleven runners who continued to race competitively were only 30 seconds per mile slower. The thirteen runners who still ran but who had let their intensity drop in training were now 90 seconds per mile slower. They were running at a similar volume, but with significantly less intensity. The VO_2 max of the high-intensity group had dropped by 1.6% – which over ten years defies the rate of ageing most other studies show. But the low-intensity group saw their scores drop by more than 12%, more in line with the commonly seen 1% decline per year.

Pollock tested them again ten years later, in their sixties, and the runners who were still competitive and had kept their intensity up saw VO_2 max scores drop by 15% or around 1.5% per year. The runners who had become 'slow, low-volume joggers', meanwhile, saw their scores drop by 34% overall and 3.4% per year. Four further studies have since shown a similar pattern and Pollock published another study in 1987 where **athletes in their early sixties maintained almost the same VO_2 max** (just 1 millilitre per kilogram per minute less) **for ten years, via high-intensity training.**[2] The message seems clear: **go fast, or go (to the care) home.**

Another study looked at the top eight finishing times at National Senior Games at distances from 100 metres through to 10,000 metres, trying to find out how fast people got slower, and didn't see a statistically significant decline until the mid-seventies. This was underlined again by another study that asked 61–67-year-olds to undertake both low-intensity and high-intensity periods of training. After the low-intensity spell, VO_2 max scores went up by 12%. But after the high-intensity period, they went up by 18%.

That study, unlike the others, included women. Science is catching up and females are less likely to be ignored now, but the general consensus in the books I've read on this is that women decline athletically a little faster with age. That could in part be down to smaller research pools or the simple fact that women often have children and/or experience menopause (as was covered in detail, by a woman, from page 48) and are less likely to continue training consistently through their forties, fifties and beyond.

Putting that discrepancy aside for now, the message is clear and applies to both genders and, though it's as yet unstudied, probably non-binary athletes too: **allowing our intensity to drop will see corresponding drop-off in our VO_2 max and we'll be allowing ourselves to age prematurely in both athletic and health terms.** Remember, our maximal ability to utilise oxygen isn't just about predicting parkrun times. Our VO2 max is a strong predictor of our healthspan and lifespan. **Fast people age slowly.**

Taking it to the max

These studies have clear training implications for masters runners, says author and coach Joe Friel, especially as most midlife athletes are starting to cut back on such workouts, he thinks. 'Maintain your weekly volume if possible, but place a greater emphasis on how hard your workouts are. Continuing to train with high intensity results in roughly half as much decline as training with long, slow distance only.'

If you train slower, even if longer, you are likely to lose performance at a greater rate per decade than if you train faster, perhaps with fewer miles.[3] 'Train vigorously, with high intensity and you'll stave off a high rate of decline in performance as you age,' says Friel. 'There may well be some good excuses for not training intensely, but age isn't one of them.'

'Am I slower on hill sprints because my muscle composition is changing, or is my muscle composition changing because I don't do hill sprints anymore?' ponders author and journalist Alex Hutchinson. 'It's not as simple as continuing to train as you always have. If you want to hang on to as much explosive power as possible, you need to move and train in explosive ways.'

Hold on, though, didn't the *Daily Mail* say running is bad for our hearts? And running harder is only going to test that worrying idea. Well, yes, endurance athletes can have a higher incidence of arrhythmias (inconsistent rhythm of heartbeat), heart scarring, myocardial fibrosis and, at marathon finish lines, cardiac troponin levels similar to heart attack victims, although they subside very quickly.

The truth is that science is still trying to understand all of these things, not least why they happen to men much more so than women. Long-term endurance athletes may experience some remodelling of the heart, but the prevalence and risk of heart attacks (which incidentally are statistically more likely to happen on Mondays, less so on Saturdays) in otherwise apparently healthy athletes as they age is 'low', according to a twenty-year study of 60–92-year-olds – which showed numerous health upsides to running.'[4,5] Meanwhile, a study of forty-five marathoners over eighteen weeks saw improved heart health.[6] Also, the incidence of arrhythmia increases naturally as people get older anyway.

A 2019 study found that there seem to be no concerning cardiovascular issues in the short term from running ultramarathons. Data collected from the finish line of the 2023 Western States 100-mile race in Californian summer heat also indicated that 'ultramarathon participation has few negative effects on cardiovascular health.'[7]

Even more reassuringly, the death rate at the London Marathon, which attracts a whole tranche of new runners, is 1 in 50,000, while globally fatalities at marathons are 1 runner in every 100,000–200,000.[8] Even then, the rare tragedy is usually explained by hitherto undetected, genetic heart conditions. If you have any signs or symptoms of arrhythmia (a racing heart, fluttering heartbeat or skipped beats), you should see your GP. Don't panic, though. Arrhythmia isn't a sure sign of a life-threatening or long-term issue. Even a perfectly healthy heart can skip a beat briefly and return to normal rhythm. Runners are more attuned to their bodies and sometimes notice arrhythmias before a sedentary person would. If running and endurance exercise is bad for our hearts, where are all the bodies, asks Phil Cavell in *The Midlife Cyclist*. Indeed, it's statistically much safer to run than to drive in a car.

However, this doesn't count as medical advice and any runners with any concerns should seek advice from a GP, especially if there's any family history of cardiovascular disease. But in almost all instances, exercise is very, very good for us. *And* it reverses ageing.

While we're myth-busting, isn't running bad for our knees? That's codswallop, too. Lots of studies have shown that runners have lower instances of knee osteoarthritis and actually report less knee pain than sedentary people, plus being a runner is linked to reduced disability in later life. So let's nip that one in the bud, too. Running is brilliant for us.

Can we run too much? If you're reading this primarily for the health benefits and want to know the minimum miles to run and still reap the benefits, the optimal dose may be as little as two and a half hours per week. Many of us love to run more often, though, because, well, we love it.

We may not get exponentially more benefits the more we run, but – within reason – we won't be hurting our health.

Speed works

Doing short intervals where we push ourselves to 85–90% of maximum effort once or twice a week is enough to reach or maintain our optimal VO_2 max. A VO_2 max effort is the highest average speed or power we can sustain for about five minutes. The idea is that by running efforts of up to that duration, with recovery intervals allowing us to hit that effort repeatedly in the same workout, we reach or temporarily surpass our anaerobic threshold, where our body generates energy without oxygen, before returning to a lower, aerobic intensity. The overload causes our heart and lungs to adapt to the demands, and over time improves our aerobic ceiling by increasing capacity and efficiency. VO_2 max intervals have been proven to also improve our lactate threshold and even our running economy, and runners could see a 5% increase in their aerobic capacity after eight weeks.

It's not vital to know our personal VO_2 max – and if we do, it's unhelpful to compare it to others – but what we can measure is more likely to improve. The most accurate VO_2 max tests are done in a sports science lab with a mask capturing our oxygen data (an expensive GPS sports watch is likely to underestimate this). However, that's probably not worth the time and cost for most runners. For a ballpark idea, you can divide your maximal heart rate (the highest you've seen in the last year or so) by your resting heart rate (the lowest you've seen first thing when you wake up) and multiply that figure by fifteen.

Alternatively, though it doesn't give a score, you can also just run at your aerobic capacity – i.e. horribly hard – for a full five minutes and see how far that gets you, returning to repeat the exact same course over the weeks and hopefully getting a little further each time.

It's easy to start an effort going all out, blowing up or fading and hopefully stabilising the effort, but we want to do the opposite. Start slightly easier than our perception of the maximum effort we can hold for that time period and gradually increase intensity as the effort progresses, so that the latter part of the effort is spent in those key physiological areas, for the best benefits. While doing so, we definitely shouldn't be able to string a sentence together and may express some memorable grunts and gurns.

We should stop intervals when we can sense that high-end performance is declining or we know we could do one more. Intervals must be 'only slightly more challenging than your estimated capacity for physical stress. You must be able to sense your physical limits and [don't] exceed them,' warns Joe Friel. 'Take a conservative approach.' Heart rate, with a chest or arm strap, not wrist-/watch-based, can be a useful gauge of effort, though it does lag behind. But RPE (rate of perceived exertion) – we have a very intelligent computer in our heads, after all – is still seen as the best way to gauge things, and we're aiming for an eight or nine out of ten.

If a runner is new to VO2 max intervals or returning to them after a significant break, they should try 10 x 30 seconds as a first session, ideally on a slight incline. These may not get into true VO2 max areas but will remind the body of the biomechanical and neuromuscular work and gauge RPE. We can subsequently increase the time spent under intensity by around 10%, using how we feel during and after these workouts as a guide. If in doubt, stick to a similar dosage as last time. **Be cautious to be consistent.**

Midlife athletes should warm up, progressively, for 10–30 minutes, which has also been shown to reduce injury risk and improve workout performance. It's commonly thought we should also consciously cool down afterwards, with easy running. Between 5 and 15 minutes of overall high-end work, not including the recovery intervals, plus warm-up and cool-down, is deemed to be enough in one bout or run for the stimulus. Recovery intervals should be around the same duration as the fast interval, to allow for a full recovery, most notably of breathing and heart rate. So 3-minute efforts require 3 minutes of recovery each (the restful intervals after which 'intervals' are actually named). To be honest, they're horrible. But by definition they don't last long and we know the amazing amount of good they're doing us.

Joe Friel recommends testing our VO2 max every three to six weeks and progressing by increasing either the number of repetitions or their duration over time, by no more than 10% at a time. Always err on the side of caution.

Over the weeks, increasing speed or power for the same heart rate is a strong sign we're making progress. To keep progress going, we can increase the number of intervals. If we keep doing these workouts over the years, our rate of loss of VO2 max should be no more than 5% per decade.

VO2 max workouts

- 10–15 x 1 minute, 1-minute recoveries
- 10–12 x 90 seconds, 90-second recoveries
- 5–8 x 2 minutes, 2-minute recoveries
- 4–6 x 3 minutes, 3-minute recoveries
- 4 x 4 minutes, 4-minute recoveries
- 3 x 5 minutes, 5-minute recoveries

Studies have shown that 200-metre intervals and 2-minute intervals both improve VO2 max.[9] More recently, the Norwegian 4×4 protocol has caused a stir with impressive results. This workout involves exercising at the highest intensity we can maintain for 4 minutes, followed by 3 minutes of recovery, repeated four times. A two-year study showed if done every week, it made the hearts, or 'cardiac structure ageing', of fifty-year-olds twenty years younger – although they were untrained athletes beforehand.[10]

Universal training theory suggests that more stressful runs, such as workouts, should have several days between them, usually of purely easy running and/or rest. Almost no coach would agree to days of consecutive intervals or especially intervals the day after a longer run. That's asking for injury and could encourage chronic fatigue or see regression. **Spacing hard workouts too close together and running them too hard are the two most common mistakes athletes make**, says Friel. A sub-mature runner might do a workout on a Tuesday and a Thursday, but a mature athlete is advised to have more space between the two. Friel suggests three days. These could be easy runs (think zone 1), cross-training or rest. For almost all athletes, masters or otherwise, one or two workouts a week is plenty and any more could be counterproductive. Because there's a different type of workout too that benefits most runners, especially mature ones.

It's never too lactate

We know VO2 max declines first and most in a midlife runner's physiology. Our lactate threshold – the exercise intensity at which a high fraction of VO2 max can be sustained, also known as tempo effort or the hardest effort we can hold for up to one hour – is the next athletic marker to decline, though it's affected more slowly and to a lesser degree.[11] Thirdly, our running economy (how efficient the body is while running) may suffer, though 'submaximal exercise economy is preserved with ageing in endurance athletes,' said one study.[12] This is pretty great news for us endurance junkies.

Our lactate threshold or turn point is the point at which lactate is produced and accumulates in the blood at a faster rate than it can be processed, which leads to fatigue and the runner slowing down. To be the best runner we can be as a mature athlete, while VO2 max intervals improve our lactate threshold, we should also be doing lactate threshold intervals, to raise or sustain the effort at which lactate can be cleared. Lactate was previously thought of as an 'acid' or waste product, but has recently been recognised as a 'miracle molecule' that's also good for our brain.

These intervals are longer but less intense, aiming to hit that area slightly below our lactate threshold. Again, our expensive sports watches may try to estimate this but may well be inaccurate. Think of it as seven out of ten on the RPE scale, an effort level where you could still speak two or three words. To work this out, we run a 20-minute time trial, then subtract 5 bpm (beats per minute) from our average heart rate. Friel recommends retesting approximately every six weeks. The idea is to cause a rise in blood lactate, where hydrogen ions accumulate and increase the acidity of working muscles, gradually reducing their power. Recoveries should be around a quarter as long as the preceding interval, because we don't actually want the ions to be completely cleared by the time we start the next one. We are training the body to process the lactate and ions better, allowing a faster pace to be sustained for longer. Simply running on hills on a weekend trail run may also be accidentally improving our lactate threshold.

Lactate threshold workouts

- 3–4 x 5 minutes, 90-second recoveries
- 3 x 8 minutes, 2.5-minute recoveries
- 2 x 10 minutes, 5-minute recoveries
- 2 x 10–15 minutes, 3-minute recoveries
- 20–30 minutes tempo effort

Economic forecast

The third key aerobic fitness area that declines with age is our running economy, which is less affected than our aerobic capacity/VO2 max or lactate threshold but will still suffer. Running economy is 'a measure of how fast you can run using a given amount of oxygen,' says *Runner's World*. 'If you can run faster than your training partner while using the same amount of oxygen, then you're more economical.'[13]

Famously, former marathon world-record holder Paula Radcliffe had a VO2 max of 70 millilitres per kilogram per minute in 1991, when she was a (well-trained) teenager. By 2003, her score hadn't budged, but her oxygen consumption at six-minute mile pace had dropped by about 15%. Her running economy had improved and she was faster.

Running economy isn't totally understood, but we think at least four training ideas feed into it, improve it or in some cases maintain it: easy volume, strides and intervals, strength training and good form. So, in many cases, runners are already working on their economy as a by-product.

Easy running aids capillary growth and slow-twitch muscle-fibre recruitment. Strides train our muscles to eliminate unnecessary movements and maintain well-coordinated control at speed. Resistance training improves the stiffness of our muscles and tendons and their ability to return elastic energy; while core training aids good technique. Short hill repetitions of 10–12 seconds led to a significant improvement in running economy, found one study. A classic workout to improve running economy is 8–10 x 400-metre repeats at mile race pace, with 400-metre recovery jogs. Warm-up drills that include skipping and bounding could also help improve our economy.

As we mature, our running economy doesn't need as much attention as our aerobic capacity or lactate threshold, but when plotting training it's worth considering whether we're doing the things to maintain it.

Going long

For distance athletes of all ages, a great fitness limiter is our aerobic threshold and that's simply improved by longer runs – 'long slow runs' as they've been traditionally called. Long runs aren't directly linked to slowing or reversing ageing but will help increase or maintain fitness by propping up that huge aerobic base we want, off which all else feeds. Easy long runs also improve metabolism/fat oxidation, engage slow-twitch fibres, help develop more capillaries, develop more aerobic enzymes (the chemical that helps produce fuel from fat), stimulate more red blood cell production (which means more oxygen-carrying capacity to the muscles) and increase mitochondria size. There are probably some mental and fatigue resistance gains, too. Long runs are a significant stress, however, and there's no need to be doing 20-milers every weekend or even every month. And they should usually be truly easy.

Hill strides are also something to consider adding into the weekly training mix, especially if you've never or not recently done them. In a 2018 study, 10 sessions of 30-second intervals (coupled with reduced training volume) over forty days led to the 10K times and velocity at VO2 max of twenty athletes improving by 2% (which doesn't sound like much but in sports science terms is significant).[14] 'For sustainable, efficient output in most endurance events, you need to be able to put out short-duration, higher-output efforts,' argues renowned US run coach and Leadville 100 course-record-holder David Roche. 'A car probably can't hold 80 mph on the interstate if its top speed is 85 mph.'

Roche believes that strides bring musculoskeletal and neuromuscular adaptations, which ultimately lead to increased power. They're usually either 6 x 20-second or 4 x 30-second, 80% efforts on a slight hill, dropped into easy runs once fully warmed up. They're not sprints, though, and the key but tricky thing is to try and maintain a distance-running gait rather than a sprinter's. 'Think powerful and efficient running, rather than using quick little strides or sprinting.' Short duration allows athletes to maximise efficient output while avoiding recovery costs from longer efforts. A moderate grade offers slightly less injury risk and is good for maximising output without unusually high or low cadence or altered biomechanical patterns.

Balance and structure

A masters athlete looking to optimise their running could be looking at a long run, two workouts, a full rest day, some easy aerobic work (running and/or cross-training) and two strength sessions (more anon) in an average training week. However, for the more mature, injury-prone or time-poor runner, that may be too much at times. Density, or how often we do workouts, is what gives mature athletes more trouble as they age, believes Joe Friel, who says **we simply need more recovery time**. 'We can generally do a high-dose session, perhaps even as hard as when we were much younger. But we can't do several of them in a few days' time. We need more recovery.'

A 2019 study found that runners over sixty report needing more recovery time as one of the effects of ageing.[15] They were also running less frequently per week and 88% were incorporating cross-training. But runners under sixty weren't running any less frequently than they did ten years earlier.

While both Alex Hutchinson and I concur that recovery seems to take longer, one study questions that. It compared recovery for two groups of men with average ages of forty-seven and forty-two after a 'high-volume isokinetic resistance exercise' workout. Their strength was analysed several times in the preceding 48 hours, and while the younger group was stronger to start out with, the relative loss and recovery of strength was the same in both groups. Markers of stress and inflammation were the same, as were subjective reports of pain and soreness. It adds to the argument that 'we feel old because we act old, not the other way around,' says Hutchinson.

Nevertheless, it's almost universally agreed that more mature runners need more recovery, to reduce the risks of injury and overtraining, or just to keep training productive rather than plateauing or regressing. The science behind recovery is covered from page 124, but it's important that a structured training plan allows for extra rest and recovery, especially from intense workouts. Joe Friel suggests masters athletes factor in more rest into their plan, the best type being a pure rest day with no running. For menopausal athletes, too, this makes a lot of sense and it may mean more flexibility, adapting to how a runner feels week by week or day by day, reducing volume but keeping intensity in the mix.

How might that look? Inserting breaks makes the density more manageable and Friel suggests we think of a nine-day training 'week'. This simply allows more recovery days – which could be short, very easy runs, low-intensity cross-training or pure rest – between workouts and a long run, which should always be spaced out by a few days anyway (running intervals when fatigued is a pretty good way to get injured).

The exact day-to-day structure will look different for different runners, but a sensible way to think is to allow two truly easy recovery days after a testing day, with workouts and longer runs both counting as 'testing'. How to incorporate strength work is discussed more on page 85, but most coaches agree it's actually better to add it to days where there's already some stress, so in turn easy days are truly easy, and this is when we actually make those crucial adaptations and get stronger. So the ideal day might be when we have a run workout too, either with a 6–8-hour gap between the workouts or immediately before or after a run, recommends renowned strength and conditioning coach Pete Stables (more from him on page 93). A nine-day week might look something like this:

Day 1: VO2 max workout in the morning + strength session in the afternoon
Day 2: Recovery (easy short run, easy cross-train or rest)
Day 3: Recovery (easy short run + hill strides, easy cross-train or rest)
Day 4: Lactate threshold workout in the morning + strength session in the afternoon
Day 5: Recovery (easy short run, easy cross-train or rest)
Day 6: Recovery (easy run + hill strides, easy cross-train or rest)
Day 7: Long run
Day 8: Recovery (easy short run, easy cross-train or rest + optional strength session)
Day 9: Recovery (easy short run + hill strides, easy cross-train or rest)

In this plan, at least two of the recovery days should be full rest days, maybe three. A 'short' run will often be a maximum of 30–60 minutes, and as ever it's really important that easy runs are truly easy (conversational pace, with heart rate below 150 bpm as a broad benchmark). Consistency is queen/king! Sometimes that means taking extra rest or reducing intensity, so tomorrow's run will be quality or even happen at all. Listen to your body when it whispers, so it doesn't need to shout.

Volume and cross-training

For a committed runner, it's advised that our overall volume should come down from what we could sustain in our prime, principally to lessen injury risk and chronic fatigue. 'Most of us on the high side of fifty either can't fit high-volume training into our busy lives or we honestly know that our bodies simply won't handle it,' says Joe Friel. He advises runners to seek out their 'Goldilocks volume' – not too high, not too low, just right for you to maintain consistent training with some quality but without getting niggles. 'If you make a mistake, make it on the side of too little volume,' he urges.

Mature runners can maintain volume by cross-training – such as cycling (which has been shown to be complementary to running in terms of aerobic capacity development), elliptical, stepper/stair climber, swimming, rowing or hiking – allowing for that aerobic base to be preserved or improved but with less pounding of the joints and stress on tendons. A study found that runners who alternated running and cycling performed equally as well as non-cross-training runners who ran in 1-mile and 5K events.[16]

We know these thresholds and key areas of athletic physiology feed off each other. We also won't be as fast as we can be without a big aerobic foundation. We won't be the best endurance athlete we can be without maximising our ability to use oxygen at the top end and pushing up our lactate threshold, so we can sustain the best possible speed endurance. So cardio is great, for health and foundational fitness. But speed is key, too. The third part of the ageless ace holy trinity is strength training.

'Some of it's in your head. You think you can't do stuff, when actually you can.'

NICKY SPINKS

Nicknamed the Queen of the Fells, Nicky, fifty-eight, didn't start running till she was thirty-four. She has since won numerous fell races and ultramarathons and set fell-running records, including for the big three rounds: the Bob Graham, Charlie Ramsay and Paddy Buckley rounds (approximately 100K each). The cancer survivor and former farmer returned to the same rounds aged forty-nine, fifty and fifty-one to set records for doubles on them. In 2025 she won the 168-mile Winter Spine Race Challenger North, aged fifty-seven.

It's in the last couple of years, really, I've noticed some athletic decline. Up to fifty-five I'm not sure I noticed much. I did a fell race yesterday and my legs and feet are shot! I'm really creaking – I'm going for a massage this afternoon. I don't know whether my decline is actually [due to] moving to Scotland, where there's not as many people to run with and not as many races, so I'm doing a lot more on my own; or whether it's my age.

Menopause was strange for me. I had a hysterectomy in 2012 and that threw me straight into hot flushes, night sweats and stuff, but without the emotions people talk about. I just got on with things. It was a bit like running through periods. You do feel different: you feel heavier and you lack energy. But I just charged through it.

In fell races I set off slower now, because you don't warm up. All the older runners I know start a lot slower, then they keep coming past you; they keep going at the same speed.

I eat more in races now, too. I used to be able to survive a four-hour fell race on five gels and a little bag of jelly babies, but now I take shedloads of sugar and shovel it in to keep the energy levels up.

You get more cautious too, because it hurts! If you've twisted your ankles loads of times you don't want to do it again. It gets harder to switch your brain off and go faster downhill. You don't want to fall. You haven't got rubber legs any more, you know; you're not quite as flexible. I do get a few more niggles. My knees never used to bother me and now they do a bit.

I do look at age categories now in races and I'm happier if they have a V55 category. It's really hard racing a fifty-year-old. It's a significant difference, like a ten-year-old racing a fifteen-year-old, but it's backwards. I'm eight years older and I'm slower than they are.

I just need to accept I won't win many races now. I've watched older runners and some drop out when they can't win. You see some really successful runners not running in their fifties or sixties. I've got friends who really beat themselves up when they can't beat their own times. But it's inevitable, isn't it? You know, there's no way I'm going to be able to do the times I used to do in my early thirties.

You still get that excitement. You're still racing. I set off in the early start yesterday and there were about twenty-five of us – it was still a race. You're still pushing really hard, as much as you can. I was racing with a lady who just turned sixty, so obviously you want to beat somebody older than you!

Recovery is different. I used to race more and recover quite quickly. I used to be able to do the summer Monday races, whereas I would just be hobbling around now. So I give myself more recovery. I take an extra day off running and have more sports massages, which I would have benefitted from years ago.

I have changed my training. I do strength and conditioning now. When I stopped farming, I noticed my core strength was less, and my posture changed. I'm doing more desk work, and I was slumping forward; I get sciatica. So I sit on a wobble sort of cushion thing at my desk.

I've always done speed work, but I do more now. I might do parkrun and a workout in a week. I do less volume overall, too; fewer long runs. That said, some weeks I'll go to the mountains and do 40 or 50 miles in three days. Because I still like proper long days out, you know, ten or twelve hours. It isn't fast, but it is nice.

I cut out the junk miles. I run on average four times a week. That would be the productive runs and then the other times I might go out with just the dogs, which could be a walk or run, just getting out and moving, active recovery, really.

I still want to do big things. I want to go for the Tyndrum Round [100K, nineteen summits] again, and in my head I'm not really sure whether I can do it. I'm starting to doubt my ability, because at fifty-eight it'll be a test. I do think some of it's actually in your head. As you get older, you just think you can't do stuff. When, actually, if you put your mind to it, you can.

I'm still doing big races and I'm looking at times really, rather than winning. I want to do well in myself, to have a good race. I managed myself well at the Winter Spine Race Challenger North last time; the tactical things I did paid off. I was quite pleased, because I took a risk in not sleeping. So I'm still learning about myself, how much sleep I can do, when to push.

I want to run when I'm in my seventies. I take my hat off to fell-running legend Wendy Dodds, because she's doing that. She's still doing championship fell races. I know runners in their eighties and they still happily race and yet they must be doubling the times from their thirties. Yet they're still really happy doing it. That's where I want to be.

To other midlife runners, I say: try not to doubt yourself. Try to just ignore the fact you're getting older – go for the same goals. And try not to be disappointed.

Joss Naylor said he did his best times in his early fifties. It must be that your head is stronger: you know how to push yourself, how to cope with things. 'I want to give up, I need to slow down', that sort of thing. Your pacing must get better as you get older. You're benefitting from the experience gained from all the years you've been running.

STRENGTH WORKS

The idea of lifting a barbell may have seemed loathsome to many runners – myself included, previously – but there are so many compelling reasons to do strength training, for both athletic and healthspan purposes. Though the potential downsides include going into a gym where there may be people more aesthetically pleasing than us spindly joggers (honestly, no one else cares what we're doing) or grunting and gurning at home, **the benefits are numerous and staggering. The risks of not doing strength work in addition to our running are also numerous and staggering.**

'All the cardio in the world won't cut it,' says Dr Stacy Sims, the author of *Roar* and an academic who is 'on a mission to help active women and their supporters better understand the nuances of the female body so that they can build strength and longevity'. Especially past the age of forty, research shows that even high levels of aerobic activity don't translate into meaningful changes in lean body mass, she says. 'The only solution is strength training, high-intensity power training – heavy lifting for pure strength.'

Left unchecked, **muscle mass declines from around thirty and occurs fastest in lower-leg muscles.** 'Losing strength may be imperceptible at first, but it's happening, and it sets you up for injury since your muscles support your joints,' says Nicholas DiNubile, orthopaedic surgeon and author of *Orthopaedic Care of the Mature Athlete*. Running doesn't build our quads, which support our knees, he says. 'Strength training twice a week all year can turn back the odometer. It's non-negotiable for masters athletes.'

Mature runners lose significant amounts of leg strength every year, even if they don't lose muscle mass as such. A 2014 study measured isometric knee flexion and knee extension strength in fifty-nine men and thirty-five women with an average age of fifty-seven. The participants were tested again almost five years later. There were no changes in their fat-free body mass, but there were significant changes in their performance in the strength tests. Knee extension isometric strength had declined by about 5% per year and knee flexion isometric strength by 3.6% per year.[17]

Regular strength training in an exercise programme is a way to maintain stride length and stride rate, and to better stabilise the body to deal with running's impact forces, concluded another study, although running alone was not sufficient to prevent the loss in muscle strength (dynapenia) with ageing. Better movement mechanics mean less overload and strain, plus better shock absorption and impact control, when we run.

Runners should be strength training anyway. It's proven to improve performance in experienced athletes, both female and male, in a variety of endurance sports. **Crucially for our age group, lifting weights improves our running economy and our speed preservation.** Done well, resistance training strengthens enfeebled tendons and ligaments. It can correct those barely perceptible but silently influential imbalances that anecdotally we all seem to have (from that football injury at school). Indeed, **strength training decreases injury risk for runners by as much as 66% and overuse injury risk by 50%**, found one study, explaining that stronger muscles lead to more stable joints, denser bones and fewer fractures.[18]

There's so much more. Two of the big downsides to ageing are muscle wastage and bone density decline, and strength work fights back against both. The fact that strength training, done well, will make us stronger seems obvious but it is proven to reduce the chances of falls in more mature people. In fact, balance at fifty is a strong predictor of our risk of falls (which as we know often spell the beginning of the end) at seventy. Several studies have found that the ability to stand on one leg for ten or more seconds without wobbling correlates with reduced mortality risk. Single-leg exercises, unstable surfaces, wobble boards and practising 20-second balance when you're putting your socks on or cleaning your teeth are all potentially life-lengthening activities. (When it gets easy, try it with your eyes closed.)

Running doesn't build upper body bone, which can slip away at a rate of up to 2% a year in women after the age of forty, 3% after menopause. By exerting a load on bones they respond positively, increasing strength. To optimise bone health, one study stated, appropriate weight-bearing exercise (such as running), strength training, and adequate nutrition, calcium and vitamin D (more on diet on page 136) are necessary, throughout life.

Strength work improves our metabolism and aids weight loss (or at least fat loss, as muscle can weigh more than fat), while muscle works our body's primary sugar regulator, acting as a metabolic reservoir for up to 80% of glucose. It stores far more glucose (300–500 grams) than our liver (100 grams), saving energy from calories instead of them turning into fat, which in turn helps prevent insulin resistance and keeps the diabetes wolf from the door. Insulin resistance and fat burning works in a cycle with growth hormone and testosterone release, increased via strength work, which in turn helps increases muscle, strength and power. **Strength exercises can also alleviate menopausal symptoms**, found a 2023 study.[19]

In addition, **strength work improves our immune system and helps the body fight infection**, found a study comparing women who did no exercise with those who regularly did resistance training, showing that the latter group had more active cells.

Strength training even benefits our brains. A ten-year study on female twins with an average age of fifty-five found women with more leg power had better cognitive ageing, even with the same genetics.[20] When we train with a heavy load over several weeks, we develop younger muscles. Scientists followed 324 identical twins and found that leg strength is the best predictor of brain health. The stronger twin in each pair had more grey matter and less brain shrinkage, and stayed mentally sharp for longer. Leg power beat cardio fitness, grip strength and self-reported exercise as the top brain protector. The reason? Your legs are massive muscles that demand constant communication with your brain.

Studies have also found that just two strength-training sessions a week may slow brain ageing by up to ten years. Older adults who lifted weights twice weekly for six months maintained brain volume in key regions like the hippocampus and precuneus areas, tied to memory and planning. Women aged sixty-five to seventy-five found that regular resistance training improved memory, attention and decision-making, and those benefits lasted for at least a year. Strength training boosts levels of BDNF, a brain-supporting protein, and hormones such as IGF-1 and irisin, helping reduce inflammation and support growth.

Better brain health is linked to a lower risk of dementia. After strength training, people had better associative memory (being able to remember things such as faces associated with names) and better executive function (decisions in everyday life), found a study conducted over two years.

Resistance training has strong longevity and age-reversing benefits and **could lower our biological age by eight years**, found a study of nearly 5,000 men and women aged 20–69.[21] Those who lift weights have longer telomeres than non-strength trainers and this elongation corresponds to 'reduced biological aging'. Another study has shown how strength work boosts our mitochondria. It's also a hormone optimiser, helping to regulate oestrogen, testosterone, growth hormone and cortisol. Apart from cortisol, we want to hold on to all of those key hormones as much as possible.

Those with lower muscle mass are at 40–50% greater risk of mortality, found a ten-year study of 4,500 subjects. A Chilean study of 1,000 men and 400 women found the same; after twelve years 50% of those in the lowest quartile for muscle mass were dead, compared to 20% in the upper quartile. **An eighty-year-old who lifts weights** (2–3 times a week for 20 minutes) **can be as strong as a thirty-year-old who doesn't**, found another. It gets better.

Muscle is medicine. Strength training is 'a type of life insurance' says Dr Mark Hyman, physician and author of *Young Forever*. Older adults with more muscle have a 19% lower risk of premature death, found one study. **Muscle reverses ageing at a cellular level.** When we activate our muscles, they release proteins called myokines into our bloodstream, which help reduce inflammation. But we need progressive overload. Yes, some planks may help with core strength and better technique for the runner, but we need to lift heavy things. A study found that muscle mass, and not BMI, was the strongest predictor of survival. Building and preserving muscle isn't optional if we want to live longer and healthier, it's simply our best defence against metabolic decline.

For longevity, we know grip strength is a rival to VO2 max as a key indicator. In one study, adults over fifty with a weak grip strength had a 45% higher risk of death. The gold standard is simply: can you hang off a bar for two minutes? Try it the next time you jog past a park with a climbing frame or monkey bars. It's time to get a grip.

So if you remember nothing else from this book (other than 'use it or lose it'), **to be the best runner you can be and to stay alive longer, run fast *and* lift heavy things.** So buy some dumbbells and turn to the next chapter.

Also, you will just feel better about yourself. The lumpy bits slowly transfer from around your hips to your glutes and shoulders; you look in the mirror and things don't look quite so awful – and, well, old – any more. Strength training 'helps our legs look a little less like overcooked linguine', says Pete Stables (more from him shortly). It may be tongue-in-cheek, but feeling better about our physical appearance brings confidence and self-esteem. It's good to start feeling good about yourself in middle age.

However, most runners find they're not nearly as motivated to strength-train as they are to run. There are so many reasons to do strength training that it feels like it's almost a life-or-death decision. If that somehow isn't enough, it's a big misconception that you need to be motivated to get started. You don't. Research shows **motivation *follows* action, not the other way around.** 'You don't always need to feel good to get going,' says self-styled excellence guru and author Brad Stulberg; sometimes 'you need to get going to give yourself a chance at feeling good.'

'Lifting weights stimulates our neuromuscular system, activating the maximum amount of muscle fibres,' says exercise physiologist Stacy Sims. 'It also keeps those high-energy, powerful type-II muscle fibres engaged, which we know are the first to go and benefit our speed.' Plus women have fewer of those to begin with.

Sims hears from many perimenopausal women who feel as if they have suddenly lost all strength and power. 'We see a distinct drop in force generation before we see any loss in lean mass.' This is thought to be due to oestrogen's influence on myosin's binding ability with actin (a weaker bond means a weaker muscle contraction) and oestrogen's anti-inflammatory qualities reducing the quality of the muscle before overall lean mass loss.

The benefits of strength training, says Sims, are nearly immediate. 'Even before your muscles get bigger and stronger, you wake up sleeping muscle fibres and develop neuromuscular connections that result in strength gains, after just a few sessions.' She urges females to lift heavy weights two or three times a week. On average, women are 52% as strong as men in the upper body and 66% in lower body, but with strength training they can become 70–80% as strong as their male counterparts. **The stronger you are, the longer – and better – you live.**

'Don't stop doing things because you're ageing.
Start doing things because you're ageing.'

EOIN KEITH

Eoin, fifty-seven, has won numerous ultramarathons with numerous course records, including the 268-mile Winter Spine Race three times (most recently at the age of fifty-two), and has set national records for 24-hour and six-day racing. The Irishman placed fifth at the 24-Hour World Championships, has represented his country at trail and mountain running, set a record for running the length of Ireland, and has placed both second V40 and second V50 at ultra-trail running's Super Bowl, UTMB.

It's not scientific, but from observation it seems we all have a good twenty- to maybe twenty-five-year running career. Steve Way and Tommy Hughes (see page 30) are good examples of that and I had a straight run of it from age thirty to fifty-two. In my early fifties, I thought, *I'm still running as fast as ever!* At fifty-three, however, almost overnight, it changed.

I can narrow it down to one event, the 2022 24-Hour European Championships. Training was perfect. I was happily doing back-to-back six-hour training runs every weekend. But suddenly, on the day, I couldn't run after two hours. Literally could not run. It was a complete energy drain. I still don't know exactly what it was. I suspect it was some kind of bug, maybe even an insect bite. I never got back to where I was after that. I lost the speed I had. And age doesn't help there.

These days, when I look at the numbers, the speed I'm doing hill repeats or tempo sessions was my cruise speed in my forties. So the pace is definitely going and there's no getting it back. You know, the effort is the same, but the speed just doesn't turn up, though it feels like it's stabilised a bit now.

My training aims have changed. I concentrate more on my weaknesses: explosive-type training, speed work, tempo sessions, all the things I hate doing! I've had to introduce things like balance work, squats and so on, strength and conditioning, things I've gotten away without doing for years. They're definitely becoming more important, just to maintain things.

I've reduced my mileage. Not because I think it will do much harm, more because there's just less need for it and other things are more important. I still do a long run at the weekends, but I put a higher emphasis on quality over quantity. That's my personal, self-coached tactic for getting older. Basically, work hard at doing the things I hate.

Recovery is way worse. God almighty! I used to recover in no time. I'd do a big ultra on a weekend and I'd run a Wednesday hill race here. That wasn't a problem right up through my forties. Now, it's a week since a race and I haven't restarted, because I can still feel it in my body. And now I have a watch to tell me it thinks I'm shit, too!

The 2022 Winter Spine Race was a demolition derby, a great example of experience and patience, just knowing things will play out, that you can only control what you can control. That was a perfect example of having the skill set to know how to get to the finish in your own best time. Multi-day ultra-racing is about survival, you know, getting to the finish line. People who make the mistakes fall by the wayside.

It has been difficult to go from the joy of racing, the joy of winning, to not doing so. Racing at the front has been fabulous. I've got a huge amount back from it. I've had to adjust my mindset, very consciously, because otherwise I'd be having a shit race. It's a hard adjustment. But you know, I'm in it because I like it. So for me it's a matter of reframing the race and what I want to get out of it. I have to very consciously know that I can't win and embrace the upsides of that.

One is less pressure, because there are no bad results any more. And you have to reframe the aims. If I'm not going to be competitive, I want to enjoy the race. So now I'm carrying a smartphone, I stop and take pictures. There's also much more running with other people, enjoying their company. One of my favourite Spine photographs is four of us [including Nicky Spinks] leaving an aid station and we're just laughing and joking away. We're having an absolutely brilliant time. We're having a really enjoyable race in a very different way. In adventure-racing terms, I call it adventure touring. So it's ultra touring, not ultra racing.

Another tactic is to focus on the actual race I have left, which is the age group. I'm still racing the other old boys, still checking how the other M55s or M50s are getting on, trying to beat them. If the opportunity is there to have any kind of competition, I'll take it!

Age is an advantage in the sense that, while I no longer have my speed, everything else is better. In ultrarunning you never stop learning. So as you get older, you're just building this huge experience of knowledge, which is gold dust. For me, it makes the races better and more comfortable. All the little things that used to cause pain and annoyance, you learn how to eliminate or control them. In my most recent race, I had two big issues and I knew exactly how to deal with them. One of the most annoying is sleep deprivation, but I'm really on top of that. You have to figure out your own tolerances and the best strategy for you. All that learning is kicking in and you're getting better, more optimised races. They've just got a little bit slower.

Being a top-level racer is an inherently selfish thing. To train for yourself and race for yourself, you gobble up a lot of resources; whereas now I like supporting other people. I spend a lot of time volunteering. I help out the Irish Mountain Running Association. I'm on the committee there, I'm the webmaster and I'm on the committee for another organisation, involved with other runners who are passionate about the sport, feeding back into the running community.

I get a big kick out of helping other runners at races and I love seeing people come and break my records. That's what it's all about. I learned that from the people ahead of me. They helped me. So I'd like to be able to at least match their generosity in helping the generation coming behind. You reframe and I want to give back. I've got skills that are useful and all this experience.

I'll keep doing my own races. Being brutally honest, I'll take winning, thanks very much. But there are still other ways to do it. You just kind of get real with yourself, accept what it is.

Online someone wrote, 'Every day, that day is your best day of the rest of your life. Stop putting things off and do them now.' And that's right. Don't *stop* doing things because you're ageing. *Start* doing things because you're ageing. And there's no better opportunity than today. That's probably the best piece of ageing advice ever. Stop putting things off. Do them today.

STRONGER FOR LONGER BY PETE STABLES

As we've seen in previous chapters, it's critical that the mature athlete engages in strength training. When performed correctly, resistance work will enable us to be the best runner we can possibly be. But, which kettlebell do we swing about, for how long, when ... and why?

Before we get on to that, a word of caution. Additional training stress in the form of resistance work could, in some cases, do more harm than good. When training with an already high aerobic load, or with a biomechanical issue, such as – and I'll use myself as an example here – a locked talus bone, adding strength sessions without careful planning can push the body beyond its capacity to tolerate or recover from the total training stress. In my case, recurrent tightening of the left calf limited running to distances under 3K, due to concern over the risk of muscle strain. The symptoms only resolved after my wonderful physiotherapist, Claire Wheller, identified the underlying cause: restricted mobility of the talus. Following manual mobilisation, the symptoms subsided completely. So context matters. To pin an injury on a single cause is, frankly, myopic. **Injuries rarely come from a single source. They tend to emerge from a combination of training errors, recovery deficits and life stress.** For runners, that could include changes in sleep, nutrition, work stress or a new baby. As we've seen, in midlife, recovery takes longer and resilience to stress isn't quite what it used to be.

There's also the role of energy availability. Many athletes unintentionally (or intentionally) underfuel, especially when chasing a certain body composition or trying to train through a busy schedule. But when energy in doesn't match energy out, the body starts cutting corners, slowing recovery, impairing hormone function and making us more injury-prone. Renee McGregor has done excellent work in this space, particularly around REDs.

Then there are those changes that come with age. We might have more responsibilities, long-term stress accumulation or just a bit more training-age-related baggage than our younger self. Old soft tissue injuries tend to tolerate less stretch before failing, which increases re-tear risk.[22] Movement quality is a big factor. If our alignment is off or our mobility is restricted, loading up a barbell won't help us move better. Instead, it might just reinforce faulty patterns. In many cases, **seeing a skilled physiotherapist to restore healthy movement is a better first step than adding more weight.**

Strength training is a powerful tool, but only if:

a) we can recover from it, and
b) our body can move well enough to do it safely and effectively.

How should mature athletes strength-train?

We know muscle mass, tendon resilience, coordination and recovery time all decline with age. That may sound discouraging, but hear me out. It's actually empowering! Because every one of these variables can be improved through training. No, not reversed entirely. But significantly improved. The key is training smart, respecting recovery and working with the body, not against it.

Is it advisable to simply pick a reputed strength-training programme off the internet, or should we go with one tailored by a local gym trainer or running coach? The answer is probably no to both. You see, most strength-training programmes are built under the assumption that lifting is the only form of training you're engaging in, which means they often leave little room, in terms of recovery, for other activities. The same issue exists with many running plans. Should we attempt to combine a high-volume running programme with intense strength work, we increase our risk of overtraining.

The truth is, runners and running coaches aren't typically the best sources for lifting advice. Why? Because they've historically tended to push the idea that high repetitions (the amount of times we do an exercise in one set) and light weights are safer and more beneficial for endurance athletes, the commonly held belief being that sets of 15–20 are good for 'muscular endurance'.

The following words probably shouldn't come as too much of a shock: Hey! You're a runner! You already have plenty of muscular endurance! You don't need more of it from the weight room. And to go even further, performing high-repetition sets in the gym (or at home) may be the worst thing you could do in terms of recoverability and force production.

Sore points

First, a primer on fatigue. We need to understand why lifting weights may lead to varying degrees of soreness. The answer lies in how our muscles work and recover. Stick with me here – after digesting the next few paragraphs, you'll never look at the little pink dumbbells in the same way again.

When engaging in resistance training, the nervous system sends an electrical signal to the muscle fibres. This signal triggers the release of calcium ions, which allow muscle fibres to contract and generate force via actin and myosin cross-bridges. While this process is essential for movement, the accumulation of calcium ions has a downside: it initiates several fatigue and damage mechanisms, which can affect our ability to both lift and run to the best of our ability, for up to 72 hours.

First, there's excitation-contraction (EC) coupling failure. Next comes the real muscle breakdown, which occurs after our workout. That's correct, folks – muscle is not broken down during a workout; it typically occurs in the hours following a lifting session.

During this post-workout period, enzymes such as calpains and proteases are released, breaking down damaged muscle proteins. This sparks an inflammatory response, clearing out the debris and setting the stage for muscle repair (technically replacement) and growth. This inflammatory response can be thought of as our second wave of damage.

Fatigue also comes from the nervous system. Peripheral fatigue affects the muscles and their connection to nerves, while supraspinal fatigue originates in the brain and central nervous system, impacting motivation and coordination and increasing perceived effort. This systemic fatigue often follows the inflammatory response triggered by muscle damage.

Here's the crucial insight: the more reps we perform, the longer our muscles are under tension and the more calcium ions we accumulate. Higher calcium means more fatigue and more muscle damage. It's a fact: midlife runners typically do not recover as well as their younger counterparts, and accruing fatigue by lifting weights incorrectly will directly impact our ability to run well over the following days – even if we think we feel recovered.

Light to moderate loads of around 10–15 reps tend to cause more fatigue and take longer to recover from than heavier sets of 1–5 reps. This is because with heavier loads, the muscles aren't under tension long enough to accumulate significant amounts of calcium ions. In fact, multiple sets of 1–3 reps at around 80–92% of 1RM (one-rep max, i.e. the maximum weight we can lift for a single repetition) have been shown to cause very little fatigue and almost no muscle damage.

If we follow the stimulating reps model, it's only the final five reps – those performed closest to failure – that fully recruit both fast- and slow-twitch muscle fibres. These are what are commonly referred to as the 'effective reps'. So, if we're doing a set of 10–15 reps, what are those first 5–10 actually doing? Arguably, not much – unless we're into bonus muscle soreness, and chasing a sick 'pump' (yes, growing up, my idols were an odd combination of Arnie and Prefontaine).

Why is it so important to recruit all of our muscle fibres? Because maximal muscle fibre recruitment via heavy, low-volume training improves the mechanical properties of muscle, enhances tendon stiffness and increases neural drive – helping to maintain force production as we age.

Strength versus speed

But doesn't lifting heavy weights make us slower runners? It can, if we ignore the principles outlined earlier. Excessive sets and reps, too much time under tension and training to fatigue can promote a shift from faster-twitch to slower-twitch muscle fibres. For the experienced runner, particularly those over forty, lifting heavy is unlikely to increase top-end speed, but it could help us maintain it. Is having more slow-twitch or 'endurance' fibres a bad thing? Absolutely not. But ageing naturally encourages this shift, regardless of what we do. Our best bet is to fight to preserve what top-end speed we still have. We're living in a new era of running, where athletes are staying competitive well past what was once considered their prime. Faster recovery, better fuelling, super shoes and, yes, strength training are all pushing the clock back.

Should men and women train differently? To date, there are no studies on female subjects that show resistance training should be performed differently to men – even during menopause. The timing of training and nutrition-composition during this time, however, is a different matter (see page 136). Lifting should be a priority later in life for both men and women. Scientists say that what is most dangerous is not lifting at all.

Sport-specific exercises

Heavy lifting is not inherently sport-specific. Instead, it promotes general physical adaptations, like increased work capacity, tendon stiffness, muscle cross-sectional area and motor unit (muscle fibre) recruitment – all positive things. These qualities are best developed with heavy loads and exercises that allow for maximal force production.

In some cases, machine-based exercises like the leg press may be more effective than barbell squats. They require less coordination and stability, reducing perceived effort and allowing us to lift heavier loads and recruit more muscle fibres. This can enhance tendon stiffness and drive adaptation.

That said, stability is a key element of strength and should also be trained, ideally with loads that are heavy but safe. Exercises like barbell marches and step-ups strike a good balance. For balance and proprioception, single-leg deadlifts and squats are excellent, though their steeper learning curve and mobility demands make marches and step-ups more accessible and directly applicable to running.

Upper body work, such as the bench press, was once dismissed as irrelevant for runners but now shows clear benefit. It helps develop upper-body strength, rate of force development and neural drive – all without taxing the legs. Remember, we're training the nervous system to better recruit as many of our fast- and slow-twitch muscle fibres as it can, as quickly as possible.

Plyometrics and isometrics

By now, we know that lifting weights increases tendon stiffness. But what about muscle stiffness – does that go up, too? And, more importantly, do we even *want* muscle stiffness? The answer: no and yes.

This is where plyometric training becomes particularly important. While plyometrics can greatly enhance athletic performance, they must be implemented with care to reduce the risk of injury. Unfortunately, it's common (especially on social media) to see 'coaches' lump basic plyometrics together with flashy but significantly riskier movements, despite the substantial difference in injury risk between the two categories.

As ageing distance runners, we need to be wary of which plyometric drills we include and the dosage, especially if we're already performing our drills and strides prior to sessions. However, for those who don't include any plyos in their warm-ups, I like to add just a touch: 2 sets of 10–15-metre locomotive pogos twice a week, right before lifting. These are known as light-tier plyos, easy on the body compared to the higher-impact stuff. Keeping them locomotive (moving forward rather than in place) improves the carryover to running.

Do double-leg pogos one day, single-leg the other. From there, you can gradually build volume, add variations and eventually move up the intensity ladder. But for our purposes here, these will do just fine. My advice is not to switch these exercises every week. Deriving the benefit we want from plyometrics takes a LOT of practising the basics, over and over again.

Now let's touch on isometrics. There are two basic types here: pushes and holds. Push-style isometrics involve generating maximum force against an immovable object, and they can mimic the benefits of heavy lifting. I love them and I use them. The catch? Without force plates or similar gear, it's tough (not impossible) to track progress. And as athletes, we like feedback. It's the same reason that doing the same strength routine on repeat, with no progression, feels dull and we give up after a few weeks. We get bored because we crave progress, like dropping 10 seconds off a 5K. Recording our weight, sets and reps each week provides simple, tangible data we can track.

What *are* useful and easy to implement are body-weight isometric holds to offload tendons before racing or help recovery post-race. Think 3 sets of 30 seconds each, focusing on the hip, knee and ankle complex, such as split squats, single-leg glute bridges and ankle holds. They're simple, practical and effective.

Home training can be nearly as effective as gym training, but adherence varies: some people thrive in social settings; others find them overwhelming. But excellent results are achievable at home with minimal equipment.

The double progression method

To make continued progress, the double progression method is an idea that helps us build muscle and improve the components of strength by progressing in two ways: increasing reps and increasing weight.

First, focus on gradually increasing the number of repetitions, such as 5–8 reps, while using the same weight. Once you can complete the top end of that rep range with good form, increase the weight slightly and start the process again, at the lower end of the rep range. This method ensures steady, manageable progress and reduces the risk of injury

For those with prior gym experience, training with low reps – as low as 3 per set – can be highly effective, as long as you're not pushing to absolute failure (i.e. you can't lift any more). Aim to finish each set with one rep in reserve, even if that means reducing the load on your second or third set to maintain that target. For most compound lifts (stressing multiple muscle groups in one movement), I recommend 2–3 sets of 3–5 reps (use 3 sets for 3 reps, and 2 sets for 4 or more reps).

If you're newer to lifting, though, build coordination and solid movement patterns first. Slightly higher reps, in the 6–8 range, allow for more practice and better motor learning. One key rule: if your range of motion shortens as the weight increases, stop. Only add load when you can maintain full, consistent movement.

If you hit a plateau – say you can't get past 7 reps on your second set – don't worry. Just stick with that weight and rep range for now. You're still making progress or at the very least maintaining your current strength. A stall like this can happen for many reasons: your current endurance training load, a drop in body weight or suboptimal recovery, among others. But if your form is solid and you're recovering well, it might be time to increase the load and reduce your reps, dropping back down to as few as 3 per set. From there, you can begin building up again towards a rep range of 6–8.

Rest periods

Rest between sets should be 3–5 minutes. Why?

a) To avoid unnecessary fatigue caused by shorter rest intervals
b) To ensure full recovery so that subsequent sets are performed at maximal effort

'But 3–5 minutes is ages to wait between sets!' I know, I get it; we endurance folk *love* to get a sweat on. We really want to feel like we've done something when we work out – the mental picture of 'that guy' sweating excessively all over the stationary bike and the adjustable bench, wearing inappropriately tiny shorts, comes to mind. I'm here to tell you that if you honestly want to improve your strength, the opposite approach is truly the path to continued and lasting progress. More rest between sets means your hard efforts will be of higher quality, producing better results. Short rest means your perception of fatigue will be higher during work sets and you risk not stimulating the targeted muscle fibres effectively. None of us fail a set because our muscles simply cannot do any more work. We fail a set because we have reached our maximum tolerable perceived effort. Rest is your friend.

Where does strength work best fit into a run training structure? Your resistance training sessions may be performed on any day of the week, with the exception of long run days. Aim to lift either 6–8 hours pre-/post-run or immediately before or after running. With all of that out of the way, here is what I would suggest for you, the Silver Striders!

Gym-based strength session

Perform this session once or twice per week, spaced apart by 72 hours. Ideally, avoid lifting the day before a hard running session. On the same day or the day after would be preferable, but not essential. And ideally avoid lifting on your long run day.

If performing twice per week, go for 1–2 working (hard effort) sets of 5–8 reps. If performing once, go for 2 working sets on bilateral movements (both limbs being worked symmetrically at the same time) and 2 sets each side for unilateral (one limb worked at a time) lifts such as the barbell march. Over time, aim to come down into the 4–6 rep range. Rest for 3–5 minutes between work sets. Exercise-specific warm-ups should be in the region of 1–3 sets for 3–8 reps using light load and common sense.

An effective warm-up prior to strength training can be as simple as a 5-minute jog, bike or row. Mobility and activation sessions are also utilised by many athletes, but these will be specific to their needs. If in doubt, 5 minutes of jogging is fine.

Main session

(First session) **Locomotive double-leg pogos** (see page 98)
2 x 10–15 metres – shallow and springy

(Second session) **Single-leg pogos**
2 x 10–15 metres – shallow and springy

Barbell march

5–8 reps x 1–2 sets each side

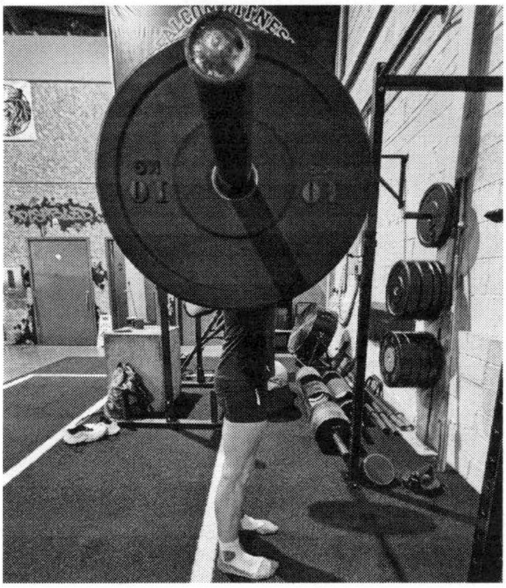

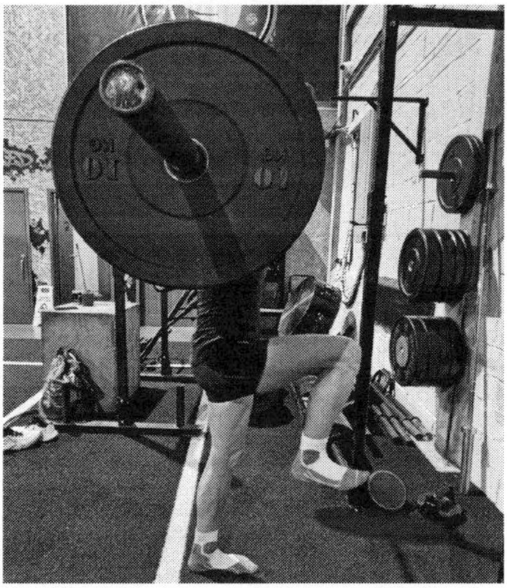

Instructions:

- Place a barbell across your upper back and stand tall.
- Alternate lifting each knee towards hip level, maintaining upright posture. Hold the high knee position for 2–3 seconds before returning to the starting position.
- Keep your core engaged and avoid leaning or twisting.

Benefits for runners:

- Coordination and stability.
- Improves hip flexor strength and dynamic balance – critical for stride efficiency and knee drive during running.

Seated calf raise

5–8 reps x 1–2 sets

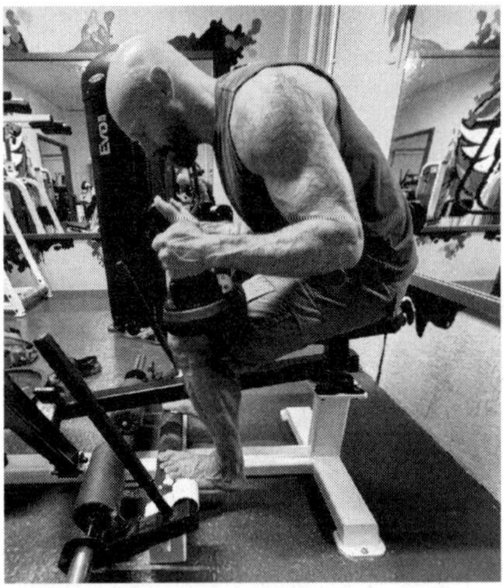

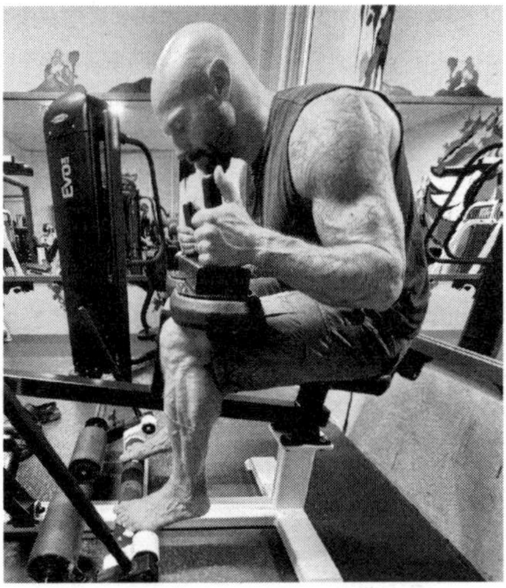

Instructions:

- Sit with the balls of your feet on the platform and the pad securely on your knees.
- Drop your heels as low as possible, holding a 3–5-second stretch at the bottom, before raising the foot back up to a neutral position.

Benefits for runners:

- Strengthens the soleus muscle, crucial for endurance and reducing the risk of calf strains or Achilles issues.

Leg press

5–8 reps x 1–2 sets

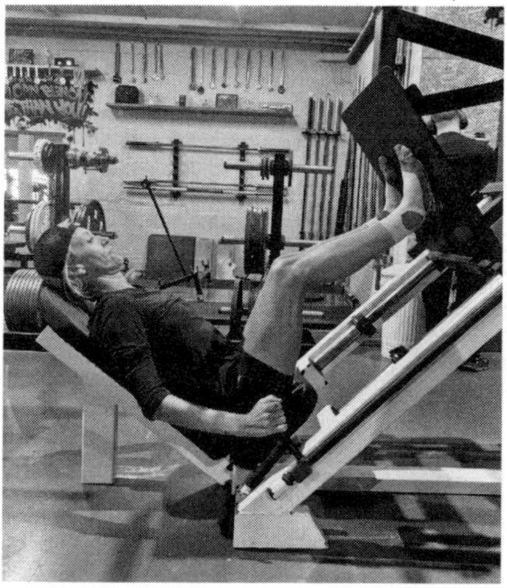

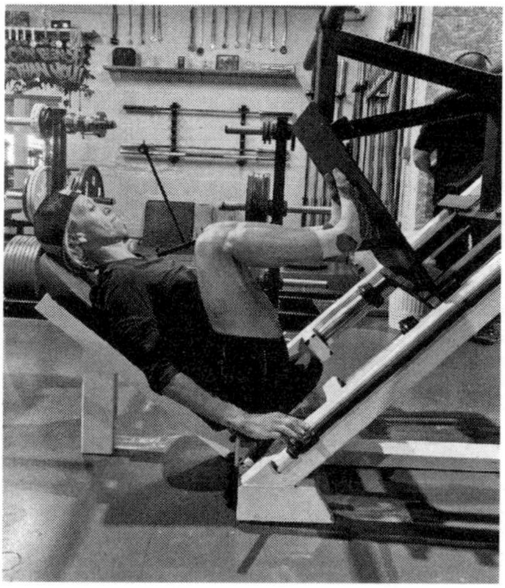

Instructions:

- Sit in a leg press machine with your feet shoulder-width apart on the platform.
- Push the platform away by extending your knees and keeping your feet flush with the surface.
- Slowly lower the platform as far as your range of motion will allow – do not force a depth that does not feel comfortable. A large range of motion is not as important as a consistent range of motion, so, find a depth you can repeat with increasingly heavy weight and film yourself side-on occasionally to ensure that the form is maintained.

Benefits for runners:

- Force production; builds quad and glute strength – key muscles for propulsion and injury prevention during running.

45-degree hip extension

5–8 reps x 2 sets

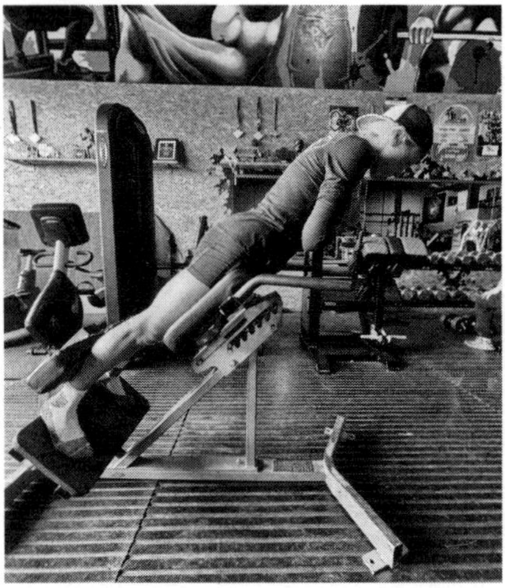

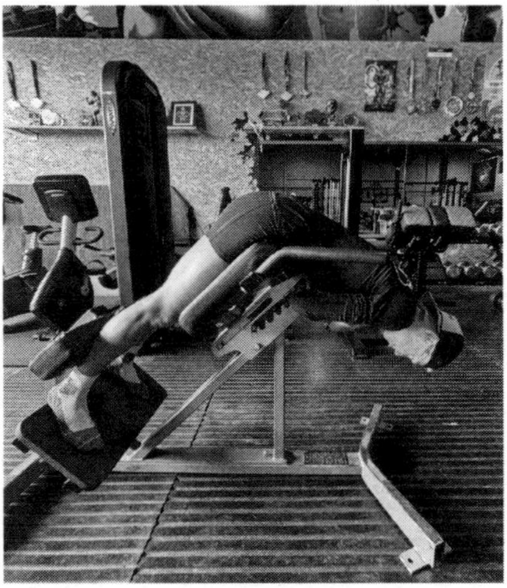

Instructions:

- Adjust the pad so it sits just below your hip crease. Your upper body should be able to move freely through the full range of motion without the pad obstructing your hips.
- Place your feet securely on the footplate and anchor your heels under the pads. Cross your arms across your chest or grasp a dumbbell with both hands, keeping your arms extended for added resistance. Ensure that your torso forms a straight line, with hips extended and the lower back in a neutral position.
- Lower your torso slowly by bending at the hips.
- Stop when your torso is at about 90 degrees to your legs. Drive your hips forward and squeeze your glutes to return to the start position.
- Avoid hyperextending (arching excessively) at the top.

Benefits for runners:

- Glute activation and strength. This exercise targets the glutes and hamstrings, key muscles for propelling you forward when running and for stabilising the pelvis. Improved posterior chain strength helps combat fatigue-related form breakdown during long runs by strengthening the muscles responsible for posture and stride control. Strengthening the glutes and hamstrings can reduce the risk of common overuse injuries like runner's knee, hamstring strains and lower back pain. Hip hinge mechanics reinforces proper hip hinging, which is essential for efficient running form and also foundational for other strength movements like deadlifts.

Hip flexor sit-up

5–8 reps x 1–2 sets each side

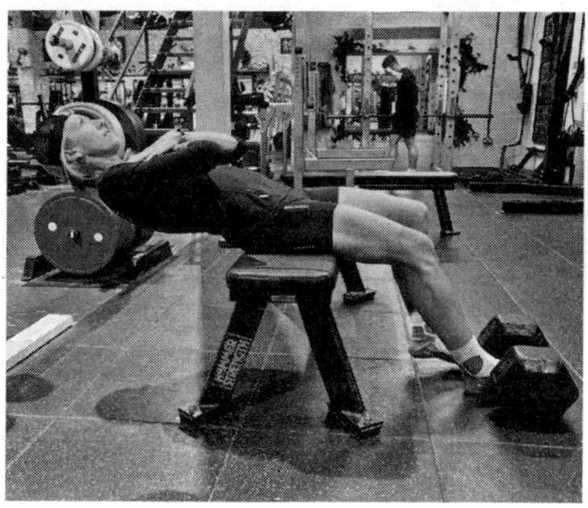

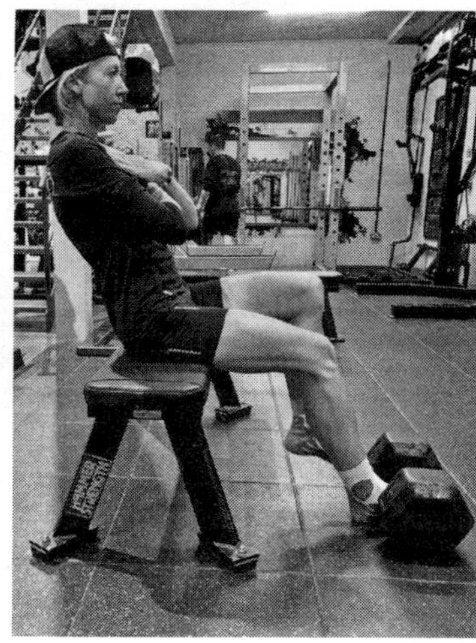

Instructions:

- Sit on a flat bench, knees bent, with one foot anchored under a heavy dumbbell. With your hands crossed over the chest or behind the head, rock backwards as far as you feel safe to do.
- Sit up by pulling the foot up against the dumbbell and flexing at the hips and waist to slowly return to the starting position under control.

Benefits for runners:

- Targets the hip flexors and core – important for leg lift and pelvic stability during fast running or sprinting.

Standing cable hip abduction

5–8 reps x 1–2 sets each side

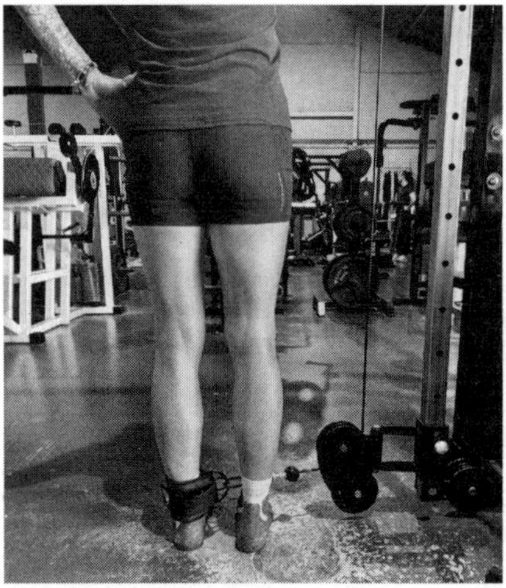

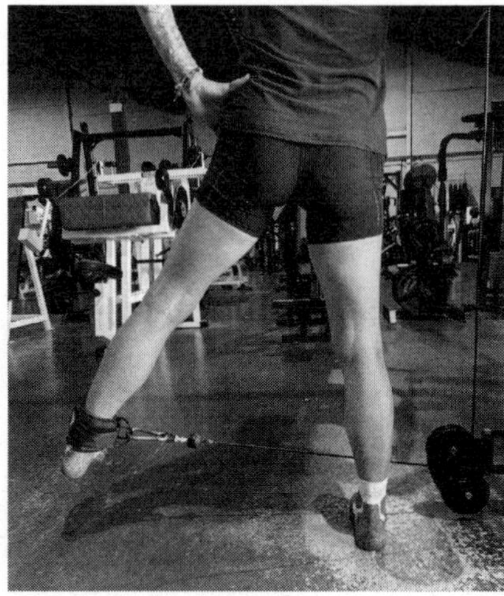

Instructions:

- Attach an ankle strap to a low cable.
- Stand tall and move your leg outward against resistance.
- Slowly return to the starting position.

Benefits for runners:

- Improves hip stability and strengthens glute medius – key for maintaining knee alignment and avoiding IT band syndrome.

Copenhagen plank at knee level

3 x 30 seconds each side

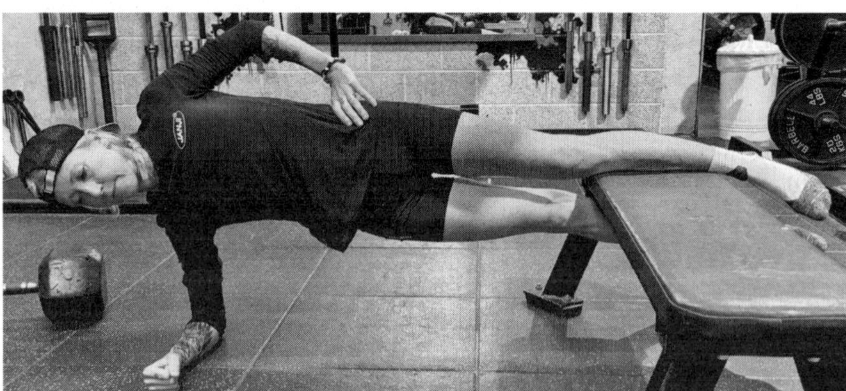

Instructions:

- Lie sideways and support your upper body on your forearm.
- Rest your top leg on a bench while lifting your lower leg off the ground.
- Hold the plank while engaging your core and inner thighs.

Benefits for runners:

- Builds adductor and core strength, reducing groin strain risk and improving lateral stability during trail or uneven-surface running.

Cable oblique twist

5–8 reps x 1–2 sets each side

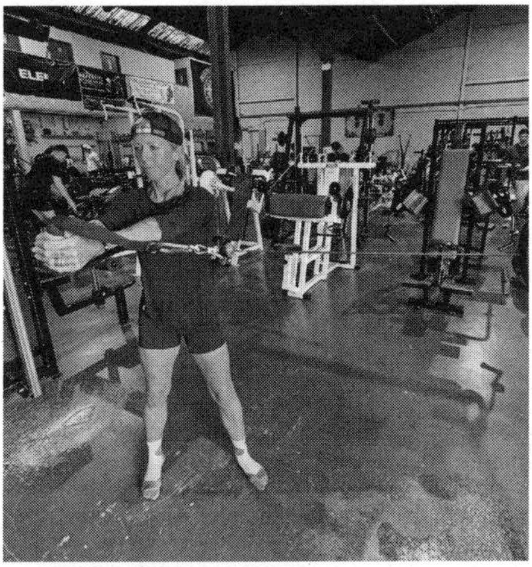

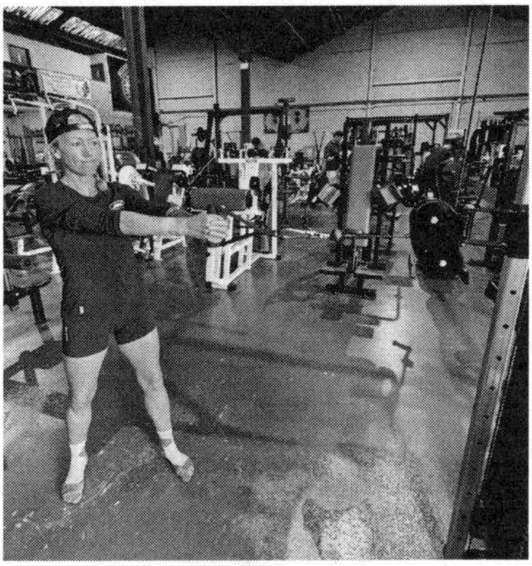

Instructions:

- Use a cable and stand with your feet shoulder-width apart.
- With your arms straight, twist your torso to pull the cable across your body.
- Engage your core and control the movement.

Benefits for runners:

- Enhances rotational core strength and coordination – useful for maintaining posture and form on uneven terrain.

Optional upper body

The upper-body lifting is placed last since the priority is to train the muscles most directly beneficial to running when you are fresh. Also, depending on how recovered you are or as a result of time limitations, upper body work can be considered 'optional' or placed on a separate day. Yes, you should absolutely train your upper body, but if you absolutely must skip any of the prescribed lifts, skip these.

Remember, if you are currently in a training block for a specific race, go for just one session per week. If in a base phase, or if muscle gain is a priority, go for twice weekly.

Seated chest press

5–8 reps x 1–2 sets

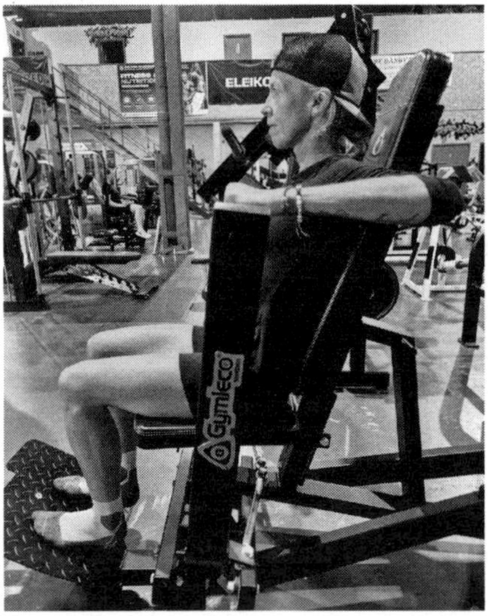

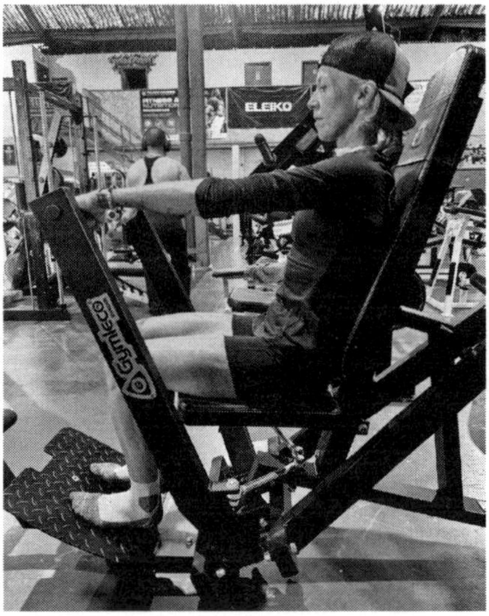

Instructions:

- Adjust the seat height so the handles are level with your chest.
- Sit with your back flat against the pad and your feet flat on the floor.
- Grip the handles with your palms facing forward and your elbows bent at about 90 degrees.
- Push the handles forward until your arms are fully extended but not locked.
- Slowly return to the starting position under control.

Benefits for runners:

- Force production. The seated chest press strengthens the pectorals, shoulders and triceps – muscles important for upper-body posture and arm drive. A stronger upper body improves running efficiency, balance and endurance, especially during long runs or hill climbs. It also helps counteract muscle imbalances from predominantly lower-body training.

Wide grip lat pulldown

5–8 reps x 1–2 sets

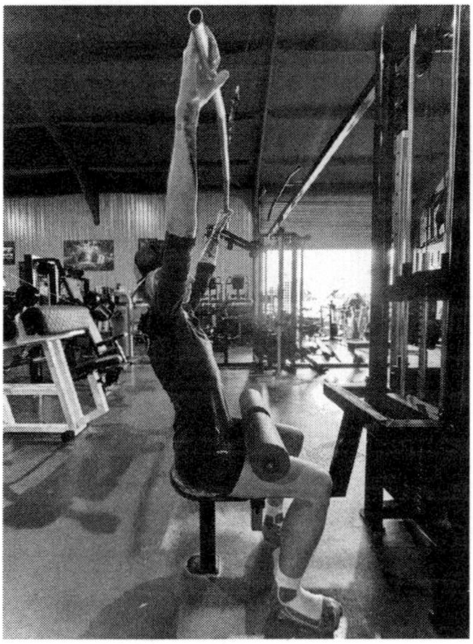

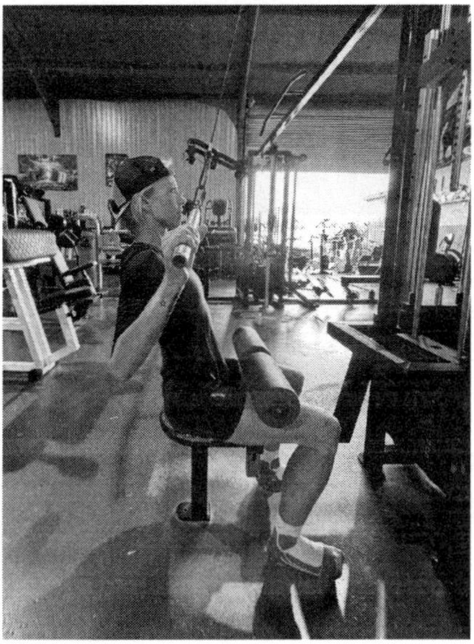

Instructions:

- Sit at a lat pulldown machine and grip the bar wider than shoulder width.
- With a slight lean back, pull the bar down to just below your chin, squeezing your shoulder blades together.
- Slowly return to the starting position.

Benefits for runners:

- Improves upper back strength and posture – important for efficient arm swing and preventing shoulder fatigue on long runs.

Dumbbell lateral raise

5–8 reps x 1–2 sets

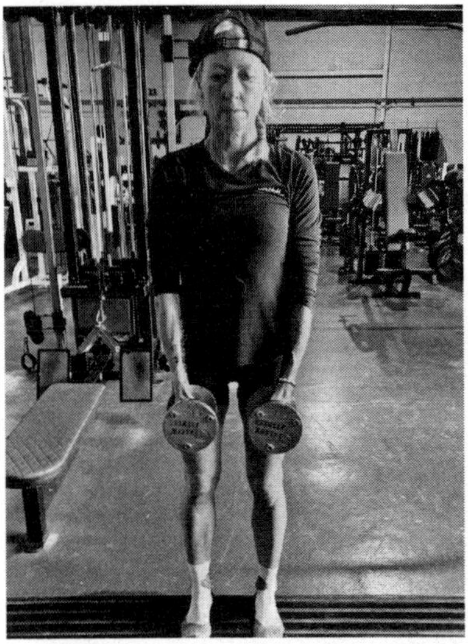

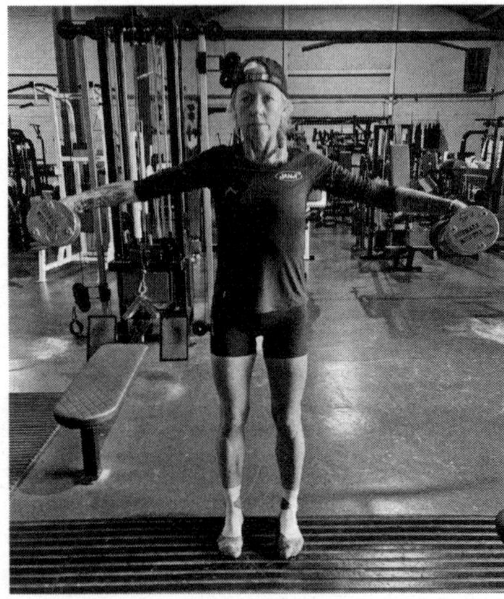

Instructions:

- Stand tall with the dumbbells at your sides.
- Lift your arms laterally until they reach shoulder height, then lower slowly.

Benefits for runners:

- Strengthens shoulder stabilisers, helping with arm movement symmetry and upper body control while running.

Home-based strength session

The following can be performed once or twice per week, ideally separated by 2–3 days. Follow the double progression method described on page 99. Minimal equipment is required to progress, but there are two essentials that should be purchased before starting:

1. a resistance band capable of supporting 5–15 kilograms of load
2. a simple gym ball

Note that for single leg exercises, the rest periods are as follows: 90 seconds–3 minutes between sides and 3–5 minutes between sets. For all other exercises, a rest period of 3–5 minutes between sets is recommended.

An effective warm-up prior to strength training can be as simple as a 5-minute jog, bike or row. Mobility and activation sessions are also utilised by many athletes, but these will be specific to their needs. If in doubt, 5 minutes of jogging is fine.

Single-leg squat to box

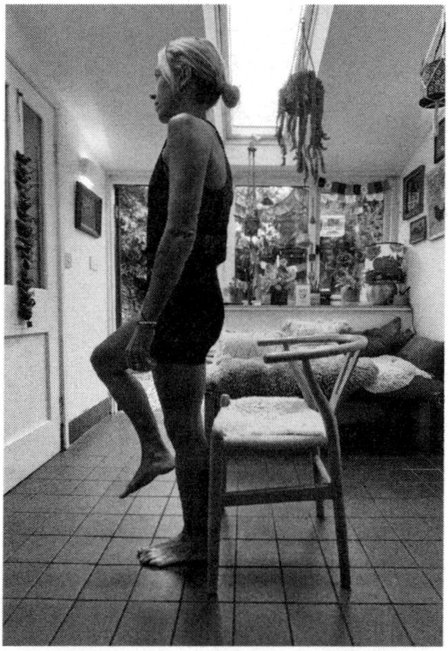

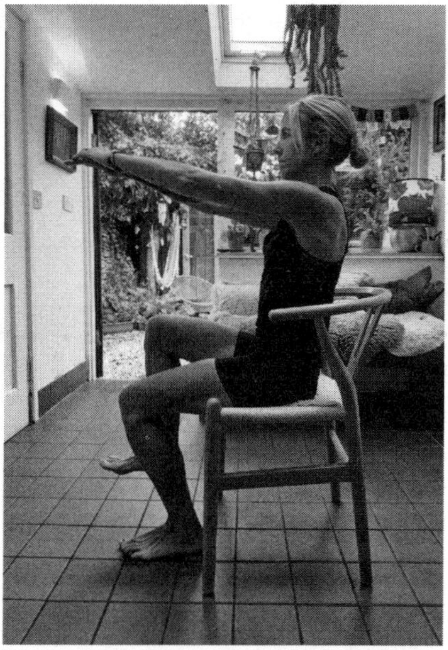

Use a box/chair set to a height that allows you to sit down without any loss of control (no plonking). If the box/chair is too low, add household items such as large books or cushions to increase the height and decrease the range of motion necessary to perform good quality repetitions. Do 2 sets of 4–8 reps each side. No weight. If you feel you could easily perform another 3+ reps during these sets, first examine your form. If you're dropping with no control, this should be rectified. It is very common to see an athlete lose control a couple of inches above the platform and end up 'plonking' down.

Maintain a tempo that, if needed, would allow you to pause at any point during the descent. Once you are able to descend over a count of four, pause on the box for 1 second and then drive up over a count of two for 8 consecutive reps x 2 sets each side; you then have the option of either loading the exercise or removing the box/chair.

Instructions:

- Stand with one foot firmly planted on the floor and the other leg slightly raised in front or extended to the side for balance. Position a box or stable chair behind you, at a height that's comfortable for a partial squat (see previous page). Keeping your back straight and core engaged, bend the knee of your standing leg and push your hips back as if you were sitting down in a chair.
- Lower yourself until your butt gently touches the box. Don't fully sit down on the box; it's just a point of contact to control the depth of the squat.
- Drive through the heel of your standing foot and extend your leg to return to the starting position.

Benefits for runners:

- Builds quad, glute and hip stabiliser strength, improving knee stability and reducing the risk of runner's knee. Mimics running mechanics by training balance and force production on one leg.

Nordic curl (with exercise ball)

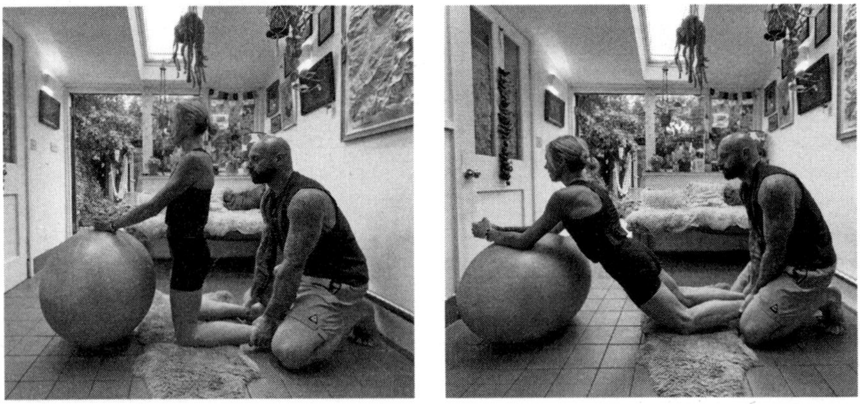

This exercise may be performed with or without a ball; however, I highly recommend starting with a gym ball if you are new to resistance training. If you decide to omit the ball, this exercise should be performed for a maximum of 3 sets of 3 reps; however, when starting, 1–2 sets of 3 reps, or 3–6 total reps, is the most I recommend. For those using a ball, 2 sets of 4–8 reps is recommended.

Instructions:

- Kneel on a padded surface with your feet secured under a stable object, or have someone hold your ankles. Place the ball in front of you, close enough to your body that you can comfortably reach it with your forearms.
- Tighten your core, glutes and hamstrings to create a straight line from your knees to your shoulders. Slowly lower your torso towards the ground by rolling the ball forward with your arms, using your hamstrings to control the descent.
- Once you reach your maximum extension (or feel a good hamstring stretch), use your hamstrings to pull yourself back up to the starting position, controlling the movement of the ball back towards you.

Benefits for runners:

- Strengthens the hamstrings eccentrically, protecting against strains and enhancing sprinting and hill running power. Using the ball reduces load while still reinforcing posterior chain control.

Nordic curl (unassisted)

Warm up your hamstrings prior to your first set. I recommend 3 x 10–30-second single-leg isometric glute bridges. Be aware that 99% of people are not strong enough to be able to lower themselves in a controlled manner all the way down to the ground when starting out. Do not attempt to do so, no matter how strong you think you might be. Get used to generating tension in the back of the legs. This does not require you to move very far. Release and drop to the floor when the tension reaches an eight out of ten. Do not attempt to pull yourself back up using only your hamstrings – hands must be used as well. Repeat for a further 2 reps.

Take your time and build up slowly. Over time you will be able to lower yourself further and further, with the eventual goal of a full, controlled rep down to the floor and then a pull back up with a little assistance from (but not reliance on) the hands. This exercise should be performed for a maximum of 3 sets of 3 reps; however, when starting, 1–2 sets of 3 reps, or 3–6 total reps, is the most I recommend.

Calf raises

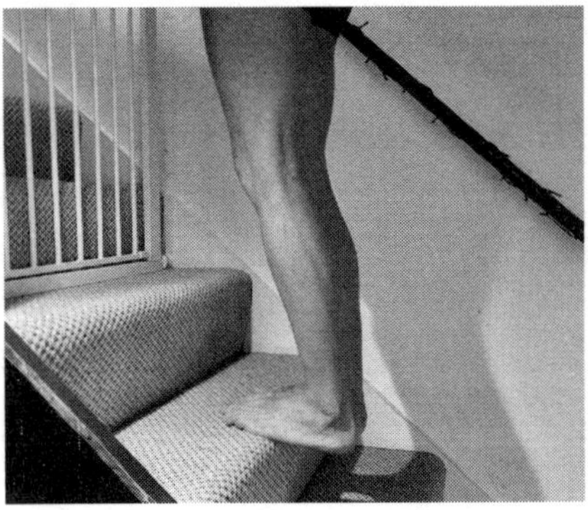

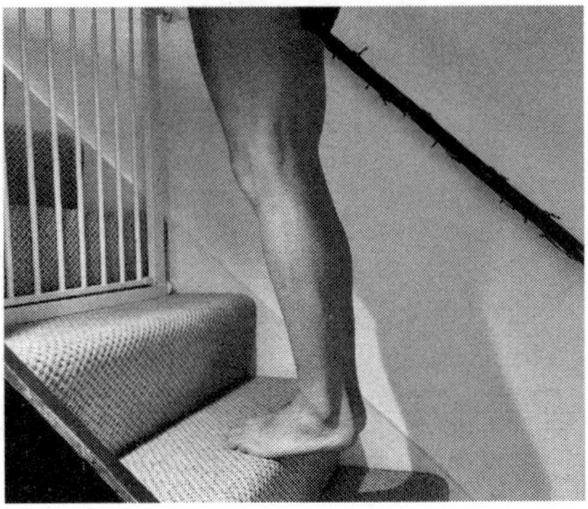

When the heels are lowest, hold for 5 seconds before pressing up to a neutral foot position. 2 sets of 4–8 reps. If this is too easy, progress to holding a load in your free hand.

Instructions:

- Locate a sturdy step, like a bottom stair, a step on a staircase or a platform designed for this purpose. Make sure the step is stable and not too high so as to avoid injury from a fall.
- Stand with the balls of your feet (the area just behind your toes) on the edge of the step. Your heels should be hanging off the edge, allowing for a full range of motion.
- Slowly lower your heels towards the floor, feeling a stretch in your calf muscles. Go as low as comfortable without causing pain. This downward movement is the eccentric portion of the exercise.
- Push up on to the balls of your feet, lifting your heels to a neutral foot position. Pause briefly at the top of the movement.
- Slowly lower your heels back down to the starting position, just below the level of the step.
- If you feel unstable, use a wall or railing for support with one hand. However, try to minimise reliance on the support to maximise muscle engagement.

Benefits for runners:

- Strengthens the gastrocnemius and soleus, crucial for propulsion and shock absorption in running. They improve Achilles tendon resilience and efficiency in each stride.

Single-leg glute bridge with hip flexion

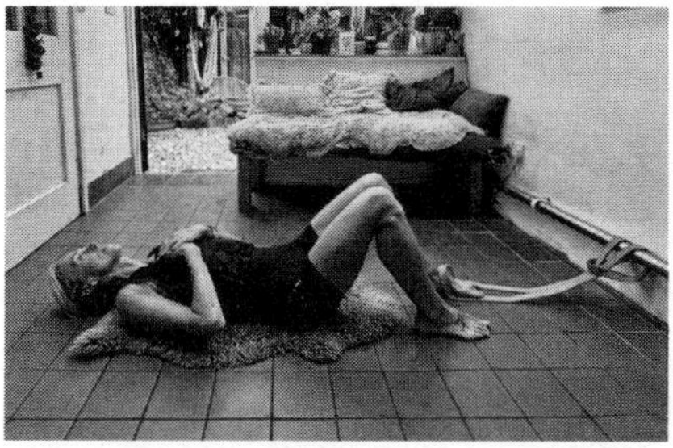

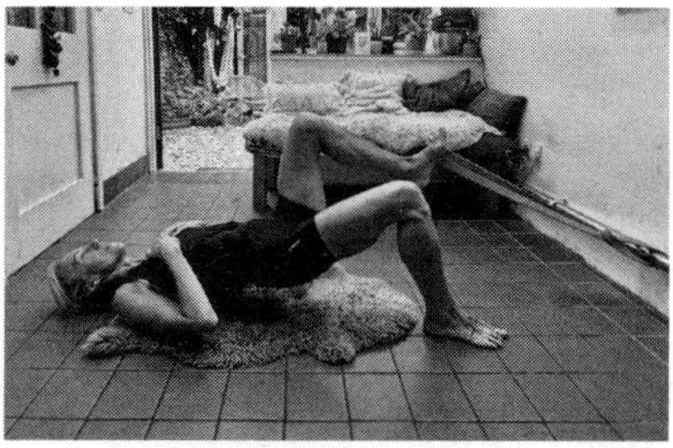

A band that can create enough tension to allow 2 sets of 5–8 reps each side is recommended.

Instructions:

- Starting position: lie on your back with knees bent and feet flat on the floor, hip-width apart.
- With a resistance band anchored to a secure object such as a bed leg and with the other end on top of your foot, lift the banded leg off the floor and extend it straight out, keeping the thighs aligned. Position yourself so that when the leg is extended, there is a degree of tension on the band. If this is too challenging, you can bend the non-working leg and keep it at a 90-degree angle.
- Tighten your core muscles and tuck your pelvis slightly under to create a flat back.
- Push through the heel of your grounded foot and squeeze your glutes to lift your hips off the floor.
- Continue lifting until your body forms a straight line from your shoulders to the knee of your extended leg.
- Maintaining this position, pull the banded foot towards your chest in a smooth, controlled manner. Pause for a count of two and then return to a straight leg position. Repeat for the prescribed reps, rest for 90–120 seconds and then repeat on the opposite side.

Benefits for runners:

- Builds glute power while challenging hip flexor stability, closely replicating running gait. Improves drive-through and pelvic control in single-leg stance.

Copenhagen plank at knee level

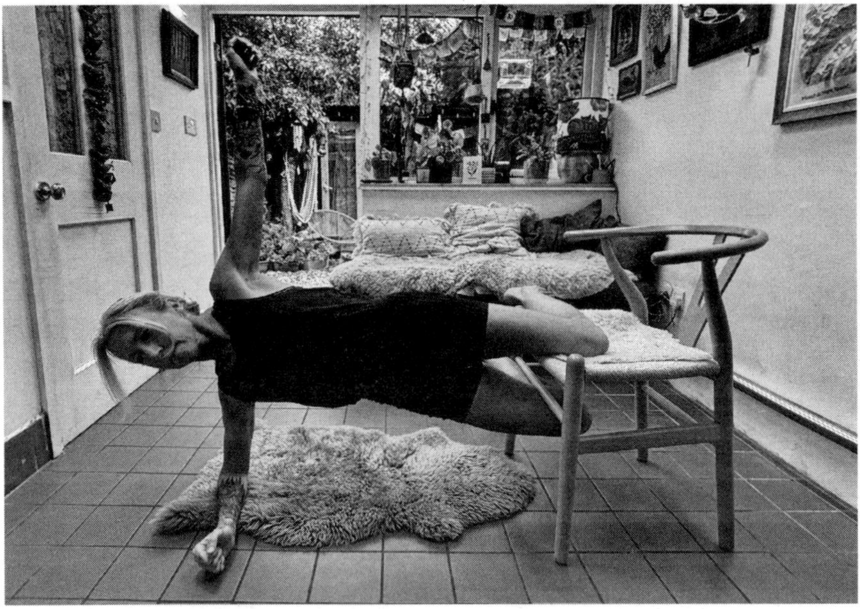

This can usually be performed with a kitchen chair, bench or something similar. The goal is to perform 3 sets of 30-second holds each side.

Instructions:

- Lie on your side with your forearm perpendicular to your body, elbow under your shoulder and the knee of your top leg resting on a bench or other raised platform.
- Press down with your top knee and your bottom forearm, engaging your core, glutes and inner thigh muscles.
- Lift your hips and bottom leg off the floor, maintaining a straight line from your head to your feet. Hold this position for 10–30 seconds, focusing on keeping your core engaged and your body aligned. Slowly lower your hips back to the starting position. Switch sides and repeat the exercise.

Benefits for runners:

- Trains the adductors and core, reducing groin injury risk and enhancing hip stability during lateral shifts in running. Also helps keep pelvis alignment steady over long distances.

Side plank with leg lift

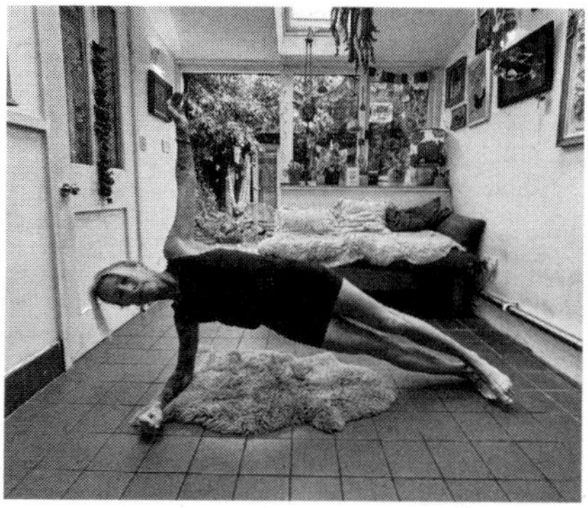

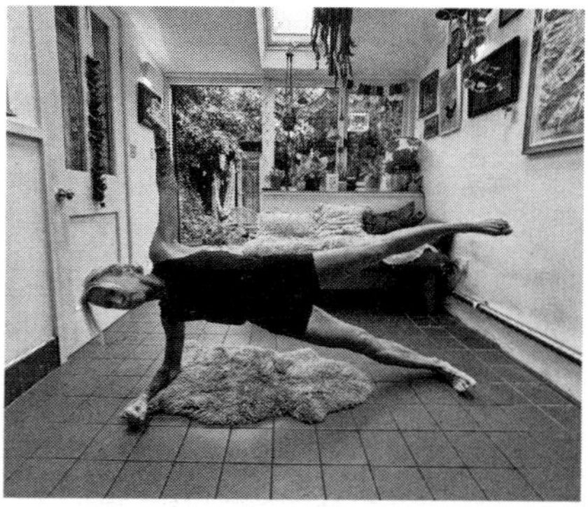

Do 2 sets each side for 4–10 reps. If this is too easy, add a hip circle band placed just below the knees.

Instructions:

- Starting position: lie on your side on a mat. Your elbow should be directly under your shoulder, and your legs should be stacked on top of each other, straight.
- Press into your forearm and lift your hips off the ground, forming a straight line from your head to your heels.
- Contract your abdominal muscles to maintain stability and a straight line throughout your body. Slowly lift your top leg towards the ceiling, keeping it straight. Aim for a comfortable range of motion, typically around 20–30 degrees.
- Slowly lower your top leg back down to meet the bottom leg.
- Perform the desired number of repetitions on one side, then switch and repeat on the other side. Do 2 sets for as many reps as you can manage.

Benefits for runners:

- Builds hip abductors (especially glute medius), which prevent knee collapse and improve stride efficiency. Supports pelvic control and reduces IT band irritation.

Table row

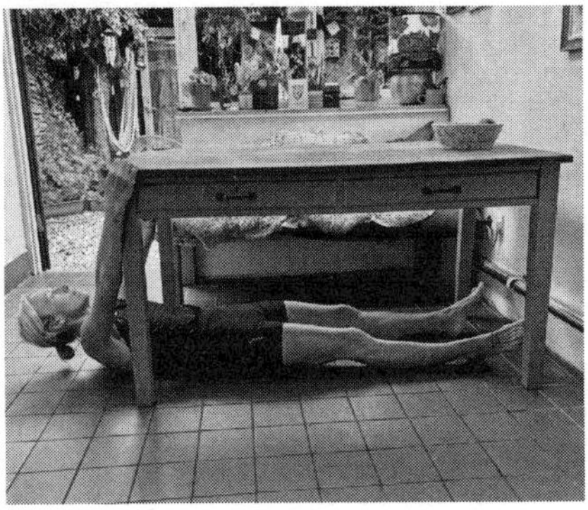

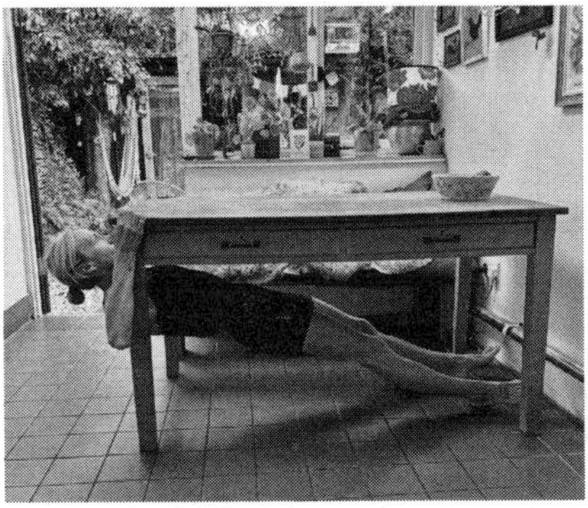

Do 2 sets for as many reps as you can manage. To make this exercise harder, try lifting one leg off the ground.

Instructions:

- Choose a sturdy table that can support your weight. Lie on your back underneath the table, so your head and shoulders are sticking out above it. Reach up and grab the table edge with an overhand grip, hands slightly wider than shoulder-width apart. Tighten your abdominal muscles to create a stable, straight line from head to heels.
- Pull your chest up towards the table, keeping your body straight. Lower yourself back down in a controlled manner, extending your arms fully. Continue pulling up and lowering down for the desired number of repetitions.

Benefits for runners:

- Develops upper back and scapular strength for good posture, aiding breathing mechanics and arm drive. Balances pressing work to reduce shoulder strain.

Push-up

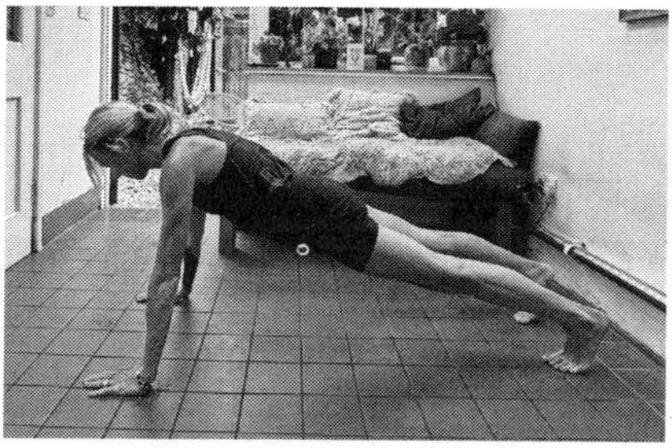 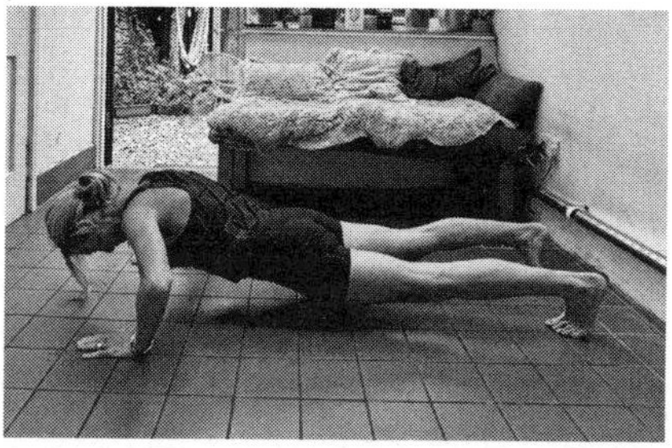

Do 2 sets of 4–10 comprising a 3-second lowering (eccentric) phase followed by either releasing the hands briefly before pushing back up, or maintaining ground contact throughout the lift. Alternatively, if you are unable to push back up maintaining a flat back, simply lower yourself slowly to the ground and finish. Come back to your knees in any fashion and begin again. To make this exercise harder, you can take one foot or hand (if you're really strong) off the ground. Alternatively, have a load placed between the shoulder blades. A small child, significant other or a heavy backpack are great options, but don't let your hips sag!

Instructions:

- Starting position: Assume a plank position with your hands directly under your shoulders, slightly wider than shoulder-width apart. Extend your legs back, coming on to your toes, and keep your body in a straight line from head to heels. Engage your core and glutes to maintain this line.
- Bend your elbows and slowly lower your chest towards the floor. Aim to lower until your upper arms are parallel to the ground or your chest is just above the floor, keeping your elbows tucked in close to your body.
- Push through your hands, extending your elbows to return to the starting position. Maintain a straight line from head to heels and keep your core engaged throughout the movement.

Benefits for runners:

- Strengthens chest, shoulders and triceps while engaging the core, improving upper-body endurance for efficient arm swing. Also helps posture by countering forward collapse late in runs.

THE BEST OF THE REST

When it comes to fitness, consistency is everything. It's not one monster workout, long run or even a week or month of epic training that bring us the best gains (in fact, that might injure us) or maintains the fitness we've worked so hard to build up. Instead, it's *consistent* training over months and months. However, as determined as we are to train regularly, real life gets in the way sometimes and athletic ageing rarely resembles a smooth curve. 'There will be plateaus and gentle declines punctuated by steep drops,' says Alex Hutchinson. You get a stress fracture, a new child arrives, a work project is all-consuming. 'But avoiding periods of rapid decline goes a long way towards slowing the midlife runner's overall slide.'

What happens if we have a training break? Research that pooled data from over a dozen studies observed that the initial effects of a training gap seem to be similar in athletes of all ages.[23] VO_2 max begins to plummet within a few days and you might lose as much as 20% after twelve weeks. These losses are down to changes in how much blood your heart can pump with each beat.

'This reduction could largely be rescued within similar time periods of training (re)uptake,' says the research, while adding that 'training reduction or cessation leads to a considerably accelerated VO_2 max drop, as compared to the gradual aging-related VO_2 max decline, which can rapidly nullify many of the benefits of preceding long-term training efforts.' Consistency becomes even more crucial when we're swimming upstream. Stop swimming and we go the wrong way faster. 'Only about half of the fitness losses suffered by endurance athletes as they get older are attributable to the passage of time. The other half can be chalked up to reduced training.'

Study data suggests that athletes who keep training at a fairly constant level over the years lose about 5% of fitness per decade – half as much as the typical non-athlete. The variation in fitness loss by female endurance athletes was 39%, while in males it was 54% (though the scarcity of data for female subjects makes it impossible to tell whether there's a real physiological difference between the sexes).

Although 40–80% of runners get injured each year, less than 10% of runners stop running due to injury, found a study of 185 runners aged fifty to seventy-five.[24] Runners in their sixties were no more likely to miss more than three months of running due to injury than runners under sixty years old, and most were able to continue running after time off for recovery.

How about if you miss a year, or even a decade – can you get back to where you were, or is that fitness lost forever? 'It probably depends on how much you trained prior to stopping, and for how long,' says Alex Hutchinson. 'There's no research to suggest a solid answer, but the risk upon resuming is that your bones and connective tissue are no longer prepared to handle a heavy load, making you more susceptible to injury.'[25] He adds, **'Avoiding periods of rapid decline goes a long way toward slowing the overall slide.'**

'I want to do races that scare me for the rest of my life.'

DEBBIE MARTIN-CONSANI

Debbie, fifty, has completed pretty much all the toughest ultramarathons you can think of, from the 135-mile Badwater ultramarathon to the 200-mile Tor des Géants, with numerous wins, including the 268-mile Winter Spine Race, Lakeland 100, Autumn 100, Thames Path 100, North Downs Way 100, South Downs Way 100 and the 145-mile Grand Union Canal Race, outright. She's also represented Scotland and Great Britain in 100K and 24-hour races and is a co-founder of Wildheart Runners community and coaching group (and producers of ace sweatshirts).

I've been running for about twenty-five years and my best years were my early forties. I won the South Downs Way 100, the North Downs Way 100, had strong runs at Lakeland 50 and the Highland Fling. A lot of people have a really good year or two and you never see them again. I feel like I had a really good ten years in the sport.

There was a massive turning point for me at forty-eight, when things like perimenopause started to show. I'm really lucky – I don't have the major symptoms most people have. But my tendons are really sore, all the time, especially this last year. It's like someone has switched a switch. I'd gone from feeling fairly sprightly, handling high-mileage, back-to-back long runs, double days, until last year.

I did Lakeland 100 and I felt really good in training, but I was two hours behind my fastest time. It's all very well saying, 'Just put your ego aside, it's different now.' But when you know those numbers in your head and you've got to still do half the race knowing you're already well behind your best time ... that was really hard. I found it deflating. I find going into races and not performing embarrassing at times.

This year, though, I definitely feel a lot better than last year. I started taking creatine and that's been a game-changer. I've done a lot more strength work, incorporating things like plyometrics. In an ideal world, we'd do everything: Pilates, yoga, breath work, manifesting. My view was always that I want to do the core things really well and everything else lay by the wayside. If I was to do it again, I would do things differently.

When I started ultrarunning, back-to-back long runs were the bread and butter. Nobody really did speed work. It was like an unnecessary evil that would cause injury. Whereas now it's really evolved and everyone's doing marathon training and bolting on long runs at the end. People realise they need to do proper speed work. Start lines now are getting younger and faster, better and stronger. It looks completely different to ten years ago.

I've been focusing more on the shorter stuff, trying to work on speed. After years and years of running at that low intensity, it's really hard to push yourself. I've been going back to club sessions. I feel like I get more out of myself when I'm running fast with others.

I've signed up for Lakeland 100 again, to get my five slates [for five finishes]. But I just don't feel like my body's capable of running a proper 100 miles right now. I want to go back and do stuff differently. I've won it, I've won the V40 and I'd like to have a crack at the V50. That would be a nice little trio. I will go into it with a different approach. I don't want to know what my previous splits are.

I also need to sort out my stomach and my nausea, which I think is a perimenopausal symptom. I've always really suffered with eating and nausea in races, but the last few years, everything comes back up. I don't even know how I finished Western States. I couldn't keep anything down. I was running on completely empty. It wasn't pleasant.

My racing mindset hasn't changed one bit from when I was in my twenties to now, at fifty. I will always turn up at a start line and give my best, regardless. I want to do races that scare me for the rest of my life – my goal has always been to run for the rest of my life. Whether I'm forty, fifty, sixty, eighty, I still want to be able to show up.

People say I smile a lot in races, but that might just be my ability to spot photographers! I think I'm genuinely quite a happy person. It's a superpower. I'm pretty much unfazed by most things and it takes a lot to piss me off, and I think that really comes into play with races that are super hard. I've gone deep into the well in many, many races, like Badwater – I honestly cannot describe how much I suffered in that race, to depths I've never been to before. I actually really like suffering.

I wouldn't ever put myself in a position where I was going to cause myself harm or injury. I've been running for twenty-five years, pretty much injury-free. I've only had a handful of niggles that have put me out for a couple of weeks, mostly accidents, like throwing myself off mountains.

I think that's because I do all my easy runs really, really easy. On my watch, I don't have pace, time, distance, heart rate or any of that. I don't give a fuck if anyone looks at my Strava and thinks I'm slow. I remember when I won the South Downs Way 100, there was a guy running with me about halfway and he said, 'I follow you on Strava – you run really slowly.' And I beat him by about five hours. I'm really, really fanatical about keeping easy runs easy and 80% of my miles are super slow. I credit that for being relatively injury- and illness-free for a very, very long time. And I will continue to do that forever.

I'm a sleeping champion. I literally fall asleep as soon as I hit the pillow. I really prioritise sleep. I think it's super important. I've been vegan for twelve years. I try to eat as well as I can, but I also have lots of chips. Because at the end of the day, I run a lot, so if I want to have chips, I'm having chips.

YOU SNOOZE, YOU WIN

To avoid injury, we know that masters runners need to be more deliberate about their recovery from running sessions. But what does recovery actually mean? Stretching, not stretching, massage, foam rolling, percussive/massage tools, yoga, air-compression legs, compression socks, recovery slippers (really?), cupping (à la Michael Phelps), acupuncture, ice baths, saunas, infrared saunas, infrared pyjamas (like Tom Brady), collagen, creatine, magnesium, turmeric, oolong tea, dark chocolate, cherry supplements, or was it beetroot? It's all a bit confusing.

We will investigate the things on that list worth looking into, but thankfully someone else has written an excellent book about optimal recovery – *Good to Go* by journalist Christie Aschwanden. She analysed the most popular recovery modalities and gadgets in 2019, and concluded that the most effective of all, by far, is simply lying down and shutting our eyes. The free one. Sleeping is training. So many good things – in fact, all the really key good things – happen when our head is on a pillow.

So much so that **we're undercutting our training and speeding up our ageing – and increasing the likelihood of diseases – if we skimp on zzzs.** Sleep may be the single most important factor in exercise recovery, according to research. Snoozing helps us physically heal, recover from illness, deal with stress, solve problems, consolidate memories and improve motor skills. Some argue diet (see page 136) is a rival as the most effective recovery tool, but many experts, including Aschwanden, assert that sleep is our number-one recovery method. 'The benefits of sleep cannot be overstated,' she writes. 'It's hands-down the most powerful recovery tool known to science. Nothing else comes close to sleep's recovery-enhancing powers. You could add together every other recovery aid discovered and they wouldn't stack up. Going to sleep is like taking your body to the repair shop.'

Sleep is the one thing that could predict running performance, agrees performance guru and author Steve Magness. Joe Friel adds that 'Chronically shortening [for example, with an alarm clock] your natural sleep cycle is likely to have a long-term effect on training quality and performance.' The old saying 'you snooze, you lose' should actually read 'you snooze, you win', concluded one study.

As with exercises and strength work, if this stuff were a drug we would all be prescribed it. About 99% of us lie down in a bed (or on a sleeping mat) 99% of night-times, but are we actually getting that critical, performance, health and life-extending recovery? Possibly not.

Sleep tends to become harder to come by as we age and it's not really understood why. Older folk tend to go to bed earlier, wake earlier and more commonly experience disrupted shut-eye. We know release of the hormone melatonin lessens, but otherwise the best scientific guess is that the ageing process disrupts our circadian rhythms.[26]

Scientists think we sleep in approximate 90-minute cycles, having four to six of these per night. In each cycle, we experience two broader stages: non-rapid eye movement sleep (NREM), also sometimes called slow-wave sleep; and rapid eye movement sleep (REM). Within these are four distinct stages of sleep: stages 1–3 in NREM, and stage 4 in REM.

- Stage 1 is a transition stage where we're in light sleep mode, which is about 5% of the time.
- We spend about 50% of sleep time in stage 2, which is important for memory processing.
- Stage 3 is deep sleep and where for the athlete the good stuff happens. Testosterone, oestrogen and growth hormone are released, which aid that crucial tissue repair and cell rejuvenation, bone recovery, capillary growth and rebuilding, enabling our bodies to make adaptations from that day's training. This is when physical energy is restored and when our immune system does its best work.

- Stage 4, REM, happens around 90 minutes in. It is the last stage of the cycle and is close to wakefulness, where more vivid dreams occur and where the brain enhances procedural memories. So for sport with motor or cognitive skills – and we can probably include trail running here – this stage is crucial. REM sleep affects our mood, memory and learning efficiency. Our brain can be 30% more active during stage 4 sleep than at some times when we're 'awake'.

When we under-sleep, we tend to skimp on REM sleep. REM can amount to 20–25% of an average night and tends to get longer as the night continues, but it only occurs for a few minutes at a time and happens more in the second half of the night. A reduction in REM sleep can lead to difficulty concentrating, and inferior memory retention and recall. People with REM sleep behaviour disorder are at higher risk of developing neurological disorders such as sleep apnoea, narcolepsy and Parkinson's disease.

Mature athletes are more susceptible to injury such as joint, tendon and muscle damage, and once soreness sets in we heal more slowly, too. So we need our zzzs. **Studies have found a correlation between under-sleeping and injury risk.** Students sleeping less than eight hours a night were 170% more likely to have an injury than their peers who slept more than eight hours, recorded a study.[27]

Another study (on men) found that sleeping for five hours a night reduces potential testosterone levels by 10–15%.[28] Five nights of sleep restriction (in this case only four hours per night) raised markers of systematic inflammation by 145%. **Testosterone drops, cortisol rises and muscle-building slows down while fat storage speeds up**, especially around the belly. Just one night of sleep deprivation reduces muscle protein synthesis by 18%, increases cortisol by 21% and drops testosterone by 24%.

Experts agree that the sweet spot is between seven and nine hours per night, with a minimum of seven hours. More sleep correlates with improved reaction times and sprint times, and feeling more alert. Our reaction time, incidentally, also includes how quickly we respond to stimuli such as strides, speed or strength work. Reaction time improves our performance and helps prevent injury and accidents. A study tested a group of twenty runners after they got varying amounts of sleep, having them perform two 12-minute exercises.[29] Researchers ran one test after six and a half hours of sleep, the other after a night of partial sleep (0.5–4.5 hours), and unsurprisingly they found that after the latter, runners exhibited a higher rate of exertion, lower physical performance and attenuated heart rate.

Sleep deprivation leads to decreased running performance and muscle glycogen concentration, and reductions in sub-maximal strength, isokinetic peak torque, distance covered, sprint times and time to exhaustion, found another study.[30] Inadequate shut-eye increases pro-inflammatory cytokines, which impair immune system function, impede muscle recovery and repair from damage, lead to autonomic nervous system imbalance (simulating overtraining symptoms), result in slower/less accurate cognitive performance and alter pain perception. We need good sleep.

In terms of our more general health, sleep deprivation also suppresses the immune system and increases susceptibility to viruses. In fact, if we sleep for less than six hours a night for around a week, we're 4.2 times more likely to catch a cold compared to those who get more than seven hours of sleep (sleeping less than five hours makes it 4.5 times more likely).[31] Poor sleep also brings increased risk of chronic diseases, especially dementia (just one night without deep sleep sees an immediate escalation in Alzheimer's proteins in the bloodstream and brain).[32]

Research has shown a direct correlation between sleep and how happy or stressed people feel, with good sleep quality linked to overall mood and better mental health. While we snooze, our badly named sympathetic nervous system (think fight or flight) gets a chance to rest. But if our natural circadian rhythm is disrupted, more cortisol (stress hormone) is released. Blood sugar level disruption from inadequate sleep is linked to pre-diabetes. Indeed, bad sleep quickly feeds into bad diet choices and weight gain. With inadequate sleep, the body holds on to fat stores, with 70% of weight loss coming from lean muscle. We could be keeping what we want to lose and losing what we want to gain. Plus we get those evening cravings for Biscoffs. Insufficient sleep leads the critical appetite hormones leptin and ghrelin to go awry, with the former lowering by up to 18% and the latter rising by up to 28%.[33] We lose the signals for being full and want to eat more, typically 200–400 kcals, show studies.

It's not just eating more, it's what's being desired: sugary snacks. Sleep influences our basal metabolic function, including uptake of amino acids and protein synthesis. Insufficient sleep the week before a flu shot means getting only half the desired adaptions. Sleep deprivation also leads to more impulsive behaviours.

Sleeping for six hours a night for a week plays havoc with hundreds of our genes, depressing those related to immunity (to cancer cells, not just viruses) and over-expressing others, which tend to be the bad ones linked to tumours, stress and metabolism. Even one night of four hours' sleep sees a 70% drop in critical anti-cancer immune cells.

Sleep shortage can blunt our desire to sleep and our ability to perceive our own fatigue. **Six hours of sleep is similar to having consumed three beers** and four hours is like six beers, found a study which tested reaction time, attention and sleepiness. Staying up all night is like knocking back ten or eleven beers. Research on pilots going without sleep found that their brains shrink, primarily the area that makes memories. *Guinness World Records* no longer includes a record for going without sleep as it's deemed too dangerous. Bad sleep is linked to obesity, heart disease and type 2 diabetes.

It's properly scary stuff. Our sleep affects pretty much everything. 'No aspect of our physiology gets away unscathed,' says neuroscientist Dr Matthew Walker, author of *Why We Sleep*. 'The shorter we sleep, the shorter we live.' Sleep isn't just a pillar of health, it's the foundation on which the pillars are built, he says. If a runner does suffer from insomnia or sleep apnoea, they'll need to seek specialist help, though Walker thinks anxiety is usually at the root of things.

Stage 3 of sleep is most altered as we age, particularly after the age of fifty, because the hormone melatonin decreases with age. Likewise, 40–56% of women going through menopause find their sleep disrupted.[34] Our proportion of stage 3 sleep compared to our youthful selves can reduce as markedly as from 18% to 3%. Sleep is commonly more disrupted and there's a tendency to wake earlier. Dozing on the sofa at 9.30 p.m. isn't at all helpful either and probably indicates an existing sleep debt.

Going to bed earlier may be the best training we can do. If we're woken by an alarm clock each morning, there's a good chance we're not getting the sleep volume our body and mind require. Matthew Walker suggests good sleep hygiene can be achieved via the following things.

- Routine: go to bed and allow yourself to wake up at the same time every day, even at weekends. Keep to your schedule – your body likes the predictability, your circadian rhythm. Wind down intentionally and start dimming house lights with ideally no big meal or liquid intake in the two hours before bed.
- Temperature: cool is better, ideally 18 °C or less. Your brain and body need to drop their temperature by about 1 °C, so they prefer a colder room. Ironically, a shower helps the body cool. Quiet matters, too.
- Darkness: block out all light and stay away from screens from an hour before bed, especially technology that makes you think about work, causes anxiety or encourages procrastination. Our devices are designed to keep us alert and addicted, masking our sleepiness (women are 10% more affected by screens). Ideally, ban them from bedrooms. If you can't manage that, Walker suggests making a rule where you have to stand up if you're using them. Bedrooms should also be as dark as possible (an eye mask helps). Darkness triggers the release of melatonin.
- Limit caffeine and alcohol:
  - Caffeine has a half-life of 5–6 hours and a quarter-life of 10–12 hours, so a 2 p.m. cup of coffee could still be in your system at midnight. That said, responsiveness to caffeine is individual and varies wildly. But even in those who think they're barely affected, caffeine could be stealing or reducing REM sleep. They wake up tired and reach for coffee again ...
  - Alcohol is a sedative, which is not sleep. Alcohol fragments your sleep, so you wake up in the night, threatening your potential to get good stage 3 and 4 sleep. Alcohol also triggers the fight-or-flight side of your nervous system. The devil's water is a potent suppressor of REM sleep.

The rest of the best

It's not just sleep. Rest, and specifically taking rest days, matters too. It's fairly standard even for most elite athletes to have one day of full rest from training. That's not just rest from running but from strength work and cross-training, too. A day off helps our body do many things. Firstly, repletion of glycogen – which burns rapidly but refills like a drip – makes low energy availability (LEA) less likely. LEA is linked to chronic fatigue or overtraining syndrome and REDs. 'Rest days give athletes plenty of time to fill up the tank,' says coach David Roche. 'With that extra energy, the body can adapt to the work that was done.'

A rest day allows our hormones to find balance and potentially optimise. Training for seven hours or more a week had an approximate 30% reduction in testosterone levels after five years, found a survey of male runners,and could suppress sex hormones in female athletes.[35] Likewise, the hormone we want less of, cortisol, is produced by the adrenal glands in response to stress, which includes most athletic activity. Chronic cortisol exposure is a bad thing and a rest day lets our body calm down.

Under-recovery stops adaptations from training happening. 'Rest days are long-term adaptation insurance,' says Roche. 'Give me an athlete that did a little bit less than they could and I'll bet they can progress more long-term than an athlete that did too much for too long.'

Rest days also guard against overtraining injuries. 'Overuse injuries are often brewing long before they become apparent as discomfort. Rest days can prevent problems before you even know about them,' says Roche.

They could also have mental benefits. 'Psychologically, rest days guard against burnout. They stoke the fire. They get an athlete ready to freaking go.' On the rest day, runners can be active with prehab or other low-stress activities, advises Roche, but no pounding of legs or structured aerobic exercise.

Stress and inflammaging

This is a good moment to talk about a word that keeps cropping up: inflammation. Acute inflammation, from a more testing run, is fine and is in fact desirable, because with adequate recovery it'll cause positive adaptations. But we want to avoid chronic inflammation, which is long-term, like a slow-burning fire that never goes out. We're more prone to that as we age and it's got a trendy, deceptively friendly, new name: inflammaging. **As we mature, what used to be a normal training load can become more of a burden and we could slip into areas of inflammaging.** It's difficult to gauge how much exercise helps or hinders this process.

From saunas to strength work, there are several examples of gentle stress tricking the body into thinking times ahead might be tough, which seems to promote our natural defences. The body's emergency response to stressors like a virus or rolled ankle is a biochemical cascade that feels like swelling or soreness, calling in key molecules for a defence and repair process. We know from marathon finish-line studies that exercise causes a short-term surge of inflammation, but the body responds with its own anti-inflammatory molecules and as we train, that response gets stronger over time. This is 'good' inflammation – as long as it turns off again once the job is done. Regular exercise is thought to protect us from inflammaging. If we train for a few months, our baseline levels of inflammation decrease, studies show; but if we stop training, the levels rise again. Because there are so many different markers, it's tricky to study and results are mixed. But older athletes have better inflammation markers than their peers who don't train. That said, younger people who don't train have lower markers still.

Inflammation is 'bad' if it doesn't shut off once a threat has been dealt with and becomes chronic or even systemic – meaning it's everywhere in the body rather than just at the site of an injury. Instead of repairing us, those biochemicals do the opposite and destroy tissue and cause cells to malfunction, accelerating ageing. Chronic inflammation is a characteristic and in all likelihood a cause of heart disease, cancer, diabetes and various other conditions we really don't want to get. In a nutshell, if we have high levels of inflammatory markers at rest, we're likely to die sooner than someone with lower levels.

Cortisol's impact on ageing is still being uncovered, but research shows a correlation between dysregulated cortisol secretion and increased inflammation, physical limitations and a decline in cognitive health in ageing populations. Cortisol initiates a cascade of physiological responses that get the body ready for fight or flight. It increases blood sugar levels for a quick fuel source, and increases breathing rate, heart rate and blood pressure to optimise circulation and oxygen delivery to vital organs and muscles, tamping down inflammation that would otherwise deplete energy reserves, slowing down digestion and even dilating pupils to improve our vision. If a hungry wolf is about to pounce on us, this response could mean the difference between life and death. When the perceived danger passes, cortisol should return to baseline levels. But with chronic stress, cortisol can remain elevated, which inhibits testosterone and potentially disrupts oestrogen production too.

Runners who push themselves hard without sufficient recovery are more susceptible to chronic stress, fatigue or overtraining syndrome. Signs include difficulty sleeping, night sweats, elevated resting heart rate, increased muscle soreness, a general sense of fatigue and burnout. We want to reduce our risk of chronic inflammation so we can live a healthier and longer life – and keep running strong.

As we age, baseline levels of several inflammatory markers creep upwards. We're not sure why exactly, but it may be because dead or damaged cells accumulate and keep triggering the immune system at a low level, or be due to gradual changes in our gut microbiome. Either way, it's bad news.

Our body doesn't know miles, it only knows stress, says David Roche. Life stress is another huge factor that will affect our running, and runners of any age are advised to keep an eye on overall health, fatigue and stress levels. Sometimes lingering stress is obvious, such as work pressure, divorce or the death of a pet gerbil. But sometimes it's a low-level, building thing, hard to detect but simmering away, doing us harm. If it becomes chronic, that means increased inflammation, higher blood pressure, a weaker immune system and worse mental health. Plus injury is more likely when background stress is high.

The body responds the same way whether it's physical or mental stress – hence why we can sweat when we feel angry, nervous or excited. The amygdala sets off our threat signal and cortisol is released. Exercise is proven to be a great stress reliever. But that means an easy 30–60 minutes rather than a hilly tempo run or 20-miler at marathon pace. Mental stress affects our rate of perceived exertion and our ability to recover, by a matter of days. Mood (e.g. grumpiness), extended muscle soreness or fatigue, poor sleep, low motivation to train, low libido, unusual difficulty in going up stairs and easy runs not feeling easy are all signs of chronic stress worth watching out for. Resting heart rate (ideally measured first thing after waking) and HRV aren't perfect science yet, but can be fairly good objective metrics for overall recovery and health. Ten points lower or higher than normal is a red flag and the most common solution is more rest or sleep and/or a big plate of pasta.

'Think about your stress (though not so much it stresses you out),' says Roche, 'measure [HRV] and find relaxation techniques that work for you. Life is hard. Sometimes piling more [training] stress on top of [life] stress makes things worse. Think long term. And be kind to yourself.'

'In the right race, I think, "I can win". I don't think about my age stopping me.'

ANNA TROUP

Anna, fifty-five, was the stroke for Oxford University's 1991 Boat Race win and a winner of age-group medals for GB at the World Long-Distance Triathlon and Duathlon Championships. In her forties, she made the age-group podium at UTMB, finishing in the top twenty overall. In her fifties, she won Lakeland 100 (twice), Arc of Attrition 100, the 268-mile Summer Spine Race in record time and broke the record for the 268-mile Pennine Way itself. In 2025, after two and a half years out through injury, she returned to win the 215-mile Race Across Scotland and the Summer Spine Race again, this time overall and with another new record. And, as I write this, she's just won the 2026 Winter Spine Race.

My journey hasn't been typical, because since my early forties foot injuries have forced me to have chunks of time away from running (I've got tarsal coalitions, which cause stress fractures – it's not caused by bone health). Before my most recent break, I could run every day. But not now.

Experts talk about different cliffs in ageing. I think there was one for me around forty-five to forty-nine. I can't just nail myself to a wall every single day now. Recovery has definitely changed; my top-end speed, too. Somewhere between my mid-forties and mid-fifties, the pace has gone.

I have to be a bit smarter with how I train. I have to focus on the right sleep and nutrition if I want to do quality sessions every day. Maybe that's another way of saying I can't be a numpty.

I don't have a structured approach to training, but I do have some rules of thumb about how many hard and easy sessions and how quickly I will build duration and intensity or mix both. I am more deliberate.

No one talked about menopause ten years ago and it happened for me without me really noticing. In hindsight, yes, there was the odd hot flush, increased anxiety, my periods becoming less like clockwork. I was working full-time, commuting, being a mum, and didn't have time to spend worrying about the odd warm night.

I suspect the training made a big difference. It's a stress reliever, which helps manage anxiety and weight gain. As a lifelong vegetarian, my fuelling pushed me towards more protein for recovery, which made me naturally move towards the sort of diet suggested for menopause nowadays. And strength work was already part of my training.

Nowadays I see every start line as a result in itself. As a younger athlete, you just assume you will get to a start line. As an older athlete, you get there if you navigate life, children, injuries, jobs. So it's a win to get there. It's a different mindset. The 2025 Summer Spine Race was the first test for my foot, post-injury. Maybe I get 10 miles down the road and my foot breaks? The aim was just to see how far I could get.

In the right race, when I am starting fit and uninjured and training has given me the confidence I need, I think, *I can win.* I don't think about my age stopping me from being able to win.

For the really long races, experience definitely comes into it and knowing yourself is key. You can race more effectively, more strategically, because you know how you can push. Experience also stops me worrying about problems, particularly if I've seen them before. I went out too fast at Race Across Scotland and was sick as a dog – you'd have thought I'd have learned! But I knew, 'Okay, I've been sick. It's not the end of the world. If I slow down, I'll be okay again.' Experience tells me I can come back from it and how to do that.

Experience also says if a course record is X and everybody is way ahead of it in the first 50 miles, the chances are the wheels are going to come off for a large proportion of the field. Experience tells me to keep a lid on those early miles.

Experience also teaches you how to train. It's almost more important than the racing, because if you haven't done the training, you're not going to race well. It's that ability to churn out the training, day after day after day. And that's probably what you saw at the Summer Spine. I wasn't being an amazing runner. I put hours and hours and hours of training in, consistently, over a lifetime, and ultimately that's what counts in those longer races.

It's a question of whether you can keep chunking out the same pace, non-stop. Because that's what I do. I just chunk it out, consistently, for multiple days, with minimal rest. Others will run harder, but they frequently can't maintain that pace, and slow dramatically or DNF.

My goals have adjusted. When my foot broke in 2022 at UTMB I was on target for a top twenty place – that was my goal. But now I'd love to win my age group. The Summer Spine Race record is breakable, the Pennine Way FKT is breakable, as is the Coast to Coast record, and I'd love to do the Winter Downs 200. I'm more careful not to do ego races now, ones where I want to say 'I've done it' but the injury risk is too high.

Talking to other older athletes, the biggest thing we feel we are up against is the time to cram it all in. It drove me bonkers when I was injured, losing almost three years while I was still competitive. Then there's a temptation to cram everything you missed into those next two years. That's what I battle with most. Because that's a sure-fire way to get injured again.

I've trained as an endurance athlete since I was eighteen, so my base probably isn't going to get any bigger. But I have limiters I never bothered to train. For me that's strength and imbalances that have arisen over the years. It's the thing most runners hate doing most. I'm in the gym six days a week and I do it before I allow myself to do any cardio. Otherwise it doesn't happen.

FOOD FOR SPORT

As we age, our metabolism changes and the spectre of the dreaded middle-age spread rears its head – or rather, its muffin top. Technically, that's due to age-related loss of muscle mass and the likelihood of becoming more sedentary as a result. That extra fat can further slow down our metabolism and our parkrun times. Too much visceral fat around our trunk area also weakens insulin sensitivity and makes us more vulnerable to diabetes.

Can we make food choices to maximise our athletic potential as we age and even extend our healthspan? Heck yes. We can do a lot, both good and bad. After sleep, diet is the second most important mode of recovery, for peak performance, health and longevity. But, especially on social media, things get so tribal and confusing, and are often simply not based on science.

'There is no question that an athlete can continue to train and perform well into their older years,' says world-leading sports dietitian and author Renee McGregor. Irrespective of age, Renee says that appropriate nutrition is integral to supporting and encouraging adaptation from training for all athletes. 'Diet, along with appropriate training, can at least reduce the severity of many age-related changes.'

As I type, a stack of books next to me includes *How Not to Age, How Not to Die* and *The Longevity Diet*; and social media is full of longevity experts telling us how frozen blueberries, turmeric and oolong tea will add ten years to our lives, if eaten in an ice bath, while nasal breathing, after fasting for 45 hours. So it's perhaps surprising when Renee says that for the mature athlete 'very little changes' from the optimal diet. The thing is, that assumes we're on an optimal, well-balanced diet in the first place.

'Meeting energy requirements and adjusting according to activity level is critical to ensure optimal health, progression and performance,' she says. 'With the current recommendations for masters athletes to maintain a certain level of high-intensity training, carbohydrate availability – particularly around these sessions – is paramount to drive the hormonal cascade necessary to support adaptation.' So let's not skimp on pasta.

Rest days aren't a time to neglect good nutrition intake, she adds, as recovery can take longer – up to 72 hours after workouts or long runs – and we need energy availability, i.e. not a calorie deficit. So fuelling rest days is equally as important as fuelling training days. Our rest days are our adaptation days.

As well as simply making us faster runners, **carbohydrates** aid bone maintenance, hormone regulation and brain function. Athletes should aim for complex carbs at all meal times and simpler carbs at snack times around and during training.

We should aim for:

- 3 grams of carbs per kilogram of body weight per day for low-intensity or rest days
- 5–7 grams of carbs per kilogram of body weight per day for days with 1 hour of moderate training
- 6–10 grams of carbs per kilogram of body weight per day for days with 1–3 hours of training
- 8–12 grams of carbs per kilogram of body weight per day for days with 4–6 hours of training.

Sugar gets demonised but is still an excellent fuel source for runners. However, glucose levels are also linked to ageing and weight gain. Sugary drinks – more commonly, high-fructose corn syrup – increase hunger and decrease satiety and consuming two per day ages the brain by two years, according to a study. **Sugar is okay and banning it is very likely to be counterproductive, but it should only be 5% of our daily energy intake.** Away from performance, try to avoid simple sugars in processed foods. If we overload our body with sugar when our muscles aren't refuelling, our body struggles to absorb it, which is commonly said to contribute to inflammation.

'There is no denying that eating non-nutrient-dense food in excess can lead to weight gain, which in turn increases the risk of these potential diseases, but there is no proof that sugar alone does that,' says Renee.

Smells like protein spirit

Protein is critical too, to help fight off age-related muscle wastage and anabolic resistance (reduced muscle protein synthesis). Athletes with good protein intake have been shown to maintain 40% more muscle mass. Without adequate protein, the body is forced to cannibalise itself by taking the macronutrient from lightly used muscles to feed more heavily used ones.

Mature runners should aim for a minimum of 1.2 grams of protein per kilogram of body weight per day but are more likely to need up to 1.6 grams, which for a 70-kilogram runner is 112 grams. Women over forty should aim for 2–2.4 grams, to aid hormone balance and weight management, prevent cognitive decline, and support muscle and bone strength.

We can only absorb so much protein per hour, though, so it needs to be spread across the day for optimal effect. No protein for breakfast and lunch followed by a whole chicken or 5 kilograms of lentils for dinner will be mostly wasted. Aim for 0.4 grams of protein per kilogram of body weight per meal (28 grams for a 70-kilogram athlete – or even as much as 37–38 grams), plus some soon after exercise and some in the evening before bed.

Consuming up to 40 grams of protein before bed can keep our body in 'muscle-building mode' for 7.5 hours, boosting synthesis and muscle repair by 22%.[36] That said, we're advised not to eat large portions in the two hours before bed, in order to maximise sleep, so experiment with what works for you.

The quality of the protein matters, too. Eggs, milk, meat, poultry, fish and Greek yoghurt are suggested, while those following plant-based diets should look to a wide range of sources such as wholegrains, beans, chickpeas, lentils and tofu – it's the combination of grains and beans that helps make complete proteins in plant-based athletes. Look to include **leucine**, an essential amino acid that acts as a precursor for protein synthesis and muscle growth. It's available in cheese and eggs, meat and fish, quinoa, nuts, peas and soy beans.

As we know, menopause triggers strength and bone-density losses and body fat gain. And muscles are less responsive to protein after menopause, when oestrogen has dropped. So female runners should aim for significant protein intake within three hours of resistance training. A scientific review of thirty-six studies aimed at examining how protein intake affects muscle mass and strength in post-menopausal women found that **those who combined resistance training with increased protein intake saw significantly greater strength gains.**

We need **fat** too, for several biological processes, and about 20–35%, or 1 gram per kilogram of body weight, of our daily intake should come from this macronutrient. That said, prioritise unsaturated fats, which are high in essential fatty acids, such as oily fish, avocados, seeds, nuts and oils. They not only help to absorb fat-soluble vitamins but also protect against cardiovascular disease and help maintain cognitive levels.

Micros management and supplements

What else will help the mature athlete delay or even partly reverse ageing? Leslie Lemon, a British war veteran who died in 2025 aged 106, believed his longevity was down to 'custard, custard, custard'. But there's a chance there's a little bit more nuance to it than that.

Magnesium, phosphorus, calcium and vitamins D, C and K are all key for bone health, says Renee. As we age, the skin's capacity to produce vitamin D – which is a hormone, not a vitamin – through sunlight deteriorates, so it is likely to need supplementation, too. Renee thinks most people in the UK should be taking vitamin D supplements for the darker half of the year as it is.

Vitamin D supplementation slows biological ageing at the cellular level, according to a 2025 Harvard study.[37] The study analysed more than 1,000 participants over four years and found those taking 2,000 IU of vitamin D3 daily preserved 140 base pairs of telomere length compared to placebo. Vitamin D supplementation prevented nearly three years' worth of normal telomere shortening.

Adequate calcium is important. That's 1,000 milligrams a day for men aged 19–70, then 1,200 milligrams; for women, it's 1,000 milligrams per day from 19–50 and 1,200 milligrams thereafter. Calcium is found in milk, cheese, yoghurt and tofu.

Potato skins, berries, oranges, bell peppers, kiwi, broccoli and papaya give us vitamin C, which also supports adrenal function and regulates stress response. Dark leafy vegetables give us vitamin K; while phosphorus is found in meat and dairy, soy, wholegrains, nuts, sunflower seeds and pumpkin seeds.

Omega-3 fatty acids aid cognitive health, blunt depressive symptoms and are associated with an increase in muscle protein synthesis. In a study of older adults with mild cognitive impairment, those with high omega-3 levels supplemented with B vitamins had 73% less brain shrinkage over one year, but both nutrients need to be present.[38] Low omega-3 is linked to lower life expectancy. In fact, one study found that a low omega-3 index had the same mortality risk as smoking.[39] Salmon is a good source, but for once supplements could be better, due to the risk of microplastic and mercury contamination common in fish.

Dark-coloured berries, extra-virgin olive oil, tempeh, dark chocolate, tea (green and black – though look out for microplastics in many teabags), chestnuts, almonds, pecans and hazelnuts with their skins on, red onions, red chicory, globe artichoke heads and olives all include **polyphenols**, which are strong antioxidants with anti-inflammatory properties, giving all sorts of anti-ageing and long-term health benefits. Colourful veggies (eat the rainbow!), fruit (especially berries and citrus), turmeric, tart cherry juice, seeds, oily fish and olive oil – the Mediterranean diet – all fight inflammation, too.

A theory behind why the **Mediterranean diet** is so strongly associated with superior healthspans is that it's mostly wholefoods, with powerful anti-inflammatory and antioxidant properties. A 25-year study of 25,000 women found that those on a Mediterranean diet had a 23% lower risk of all-cause mortality.[40]

Dark leafy greens, especially broccoli and kale, help detoxify pollutants via **sulforaphane**, which gets activated when we chew. They're also high in magnesium, which prevents DNA damage and lowers cancer risk. Indeed, **magnesium deficiency is very common in older adults** and is linked to inflammaging. Other foods high in magnesium include green vegetables, avocados, legumes, nuts and seeds, whole cereals, pseudocereals such as quinoa and buckwheat, cocoa and bananas.

Watermelon, nuts, rosemary, berries (especially grapes and blueberries before bedtime), turmeric, garlic, ginger, dark chocolate, oolong tea and doubtless many other things have been linked with age-slowing or reversing properties. The remarkable *How Not to Age* (a follow-up to *How Not to Die*) is 714 pages of nutrition advice to extend your healthspan, largely supporting the argument for plant-based foods. But the phrase 'killing yourself to stay alive' starts to feel pertinent, and as with training we can sometimes overlook the fundamentals by getting seduced by the latest new thing with only very marginal gains. Eating nuts, seeds, herbs and spices is an easy tweak that should bring benefits – 3% of total energy intake from nuts and seeds makes us one year 'younger' by telomere length – along with more fruit, veg and high fibre (such as oats, brown rice, whole wheat and quinoa), which are nutrient-dense, improve insulin sensitivity and glucose metabolism, slow food absorption and may reduce inflammation.

Should we be taking any supplements (along with vitamin D)? **Collagen** supplements are likely to benefit the mature runner, helping with joint, ligament and tendon health, and improving force and explosive movement by making tendons and muscles 'stiffer'. Like most things, collagen declines with age and we lose that explosiveness or power. Collagen doesn't seem to work for up to 30% of people, but Renee suggests a dose of 5–10 grams of bovine collagen, which may improve sprint performance and muscle gain for mature runners. Neither tendons nor muscles get any bigger, and nor does maximum strength, but the elastic stiffness of both muscle and tendon increases, according to a 2025 study.[41] Collagen is also thought to improve hair and nail health.

Creatine is getting a lot of press right now. While a number of studies support its use in sports and disciplines that involve repeated sprints or repetitive movements, such as football and gymnastics, there is no real evidence for the use of creatine in endurance sports, says Renee. More recently, there have been some emerging studies suggesting benefits with regard to maintaining muscle mass, especially in perimenopausal women. 'But on closer examination of these studies, it's clear that the inclusion of resistance training has more of a positive influence than creatine. So while the studies are promising, we still need more robust studies on protocols and dosage to warrant the use.'

Iron is important, however, and commonly insufficient in runners, though overconsumption can lead to issues too, so it's something to check with a blood test. **Cherry juice** in the evening may enhance our melatonin levels and encourage better quality sleep.

We're increasingly learning that our **gut microbiome** is really important, almost a second brain. It synthesises vitamins, influences the release of hormones including cortisol and testosterone, and helps regulate our appetite, sending signals to the brain about energy storage, metabolism adjustments, insulin sensitivity and hunger levels. It may calm age-related inflammation (that word again) and keep oxidative stress in check. About 70% of our immune health comes from our gut.

A high-fibre diet rich in colourful fruits, vegetables, legumes and wholegrains increases the desired bacterial diversity, says Renee. 'While our body can't digest a high-fibre diet, certain bacteria in our gut can, and this stimulates their growth, resulting in an improved environment', she says.

Fermented foods are beneficial, including yoghurt, sauerkraut, kombucha, kefir and tempeh. 'It has been found that including more of these foods enhances the function of the microbiome by reducing the abundance of disease-causing bacteria in the intestines.'

Probiotic supplements can aid microbial diversity, too. Probiotics are live microorganisms, usually bacteria, that provide a specific health benefit. 'They work on the principle of colonising the gut and benefit health by changing the overall composition of the microbiome and supporting metabolism,' says Renee. 'While they can be consumed daily, probiotics have been found to be most effective in restoring the microbiome to a healthy state after it has been compromised. Care needs to be taken when using probiotic supplements as most are destroyed by stomach acid and so don't make it as far as the gut. That said, one example of a food supplement that does work is Symprove. This live culture is water-based, which means it can pass through the stomach unaffected and be transported into the gut, where it can then go on to colonise and benefit its host.'

Just you weight

Let's look at the tricky subject of body weight. Ageing brings metabolism changes and Joe Friel thinks the biggest issue for the mature athlete, aside from decreased aerobic capacity and shrinking muscles, is increased body fat. Increased weight means slower running, because our VO_2 max is a direct calculation of oxygen uptake per kilogram of body weight. If you gain weight, the primary muscles responsible for powering you along have to work harder just to maintain the same pace you were capable of at a previous, lower body weight. So your VO_2 max and speed drop, accelerating ageing. 'The bottom line is,' says Friel, 'if your sport is dependent on performance relative to gravity, then gaining weight is likely a problem.' Muscle weighs more than fat, so girth measurements are a better sign of changing body composition than what the scales say.

What can we do? Firstly, Friel suggests, while the exact physiological processes aren't certain, we might have been able to outrun a bad diet as a younger athlete, but it seems to catch up with us. (Indeed, despite no significant changes in mine over the last four years since becoming an Annoying Vegan, high cholesterol markers were detected in two recent blood tests.) Even if this isn't the case for you, **consider whether there are obvious bad-faith items that could be trimmed from your diet** – it's proven to be more effective to reduce things rather than ban them. As well as sugary drinks and biscuits (high in both sugar and saturated fats), alcohol (more anon) is an obvious one, along with takeaways and ultra-processed foods, the latter two tending to be unhealthily high in sugar, salt and fat.

Ultra-processed food (UPF) is a fairly new concept and the exact health implications are debatable, but it can be defined as having ingredients mostly of exclusive industrial use, typically created by a series of industrial techniques and processes. Or, more simply, ingredients you might not find in your kitchen cupboard – for example, additives, emulsifiers or stabilisers. Not all UPF is bad for us, though. A diet containing UPFs high in fibre, such as wholegrain supermarket bread and baked beans, can be just as healthy as a 'whole diet'. The issue with UPFs is when they don't provide any nutrient value.

The UK government's generic advice for a healthy diet for most people is to cut down on saturated fat, sugar and salt, and eat more vegetables and fibre. Saturated fat and sugar directly impair the hippocampus, the brain's navigation and memory centre.

Not so fast

Fasting and deliberate calorie restriction are popular ideas in the longevity cult. Research suggests that extending an overnight fast may improve metabolism, aid cellular repair and perhaps even prolong life – though most of that research has been done on animals. In a 2015 study on humans, the ratio of 'good' cholesterol to 'bad' cholesterol had increased, molecules associated with tumour formation were reduced by around 25% and levels of insulin resistance fell by nearly 40%. However, some of those benefits may simply have come from weight loss.

Typically, fasters try to leave a gap of 12–16 hours without food. However, a large-scale study of more than 19,000 adults compared people who restricted their eating to a period of less than 8 hours a day and those who ate across 12–14 hours. The former group had a 135% higher risk of dying from cardiovascular disease.[42] There could also be a risk for bone health. We also know fasting is an ineffective tactic for weight loss.

It sounds plausible that we runners might get some of the above benefits anyway, towards the end of those long runs where we left our gels at home. There's a strong link between fasting and hormonal dysfunction (increased cortisol – which can be increased by dehydration too), menstrual dysfunction, metabolic disturbances, impaired performance and fewer muscle adaptations in female athletes. The risks just don't seem worth it. **Fasting will likely not make us faster.**

Chronic under-fuelling is linked to a cascade of negatives. Low energy availability (LEA) occurs when an athlete's calorie intake doesn't match their energy expenditure and increases injury risk by 4.5 times in women. Other potential issues include REDs, hormone imbalances (LEA is strongly linked to low testosterone in men), reduced training response, plateauing, regressing and simply not being the best athlete we could be, with the risk of more serious, long-term health outcomes. A study at Boston Marathon found that runners with LEA had twice the risk of requiring medical support and 2.8 times the risk of a major medical encounter, as well as slower performances. The research found that 42% of female runners and 18% of male runners had LEA indicators.

Lighter is not always better, certainly not in the long term, and calorie restriction can easily lead to losing muscle rather than fat. Lighter often isn't stronger either and we naturally have different body types. Studies have shown that if we fuel it adequately while training, our body is clever enough to find the right weight and body composition for us as individuals.

Strength training is an effective weight-loss strategy, says Stacy Sims, as it's key for mobilising abdominal fat, creating more lean mass and increasing the amount of cross talk between skeletal muscle and stored fat, through myokines.

However, if you know for certain your body is carrying a little bit extra, try these options:

- Strength-train – with additional protein to support it.
- Have a big breakfast, with a sizeable helping of protein, so you start the day satiated and less likely to snack.
- When you do snack, prioritise nuts and fruit, instead of crisps, chocolate or sugary drinks.
- In main meals, reduce carbs a little and increase protein, to feel more satiated.
- Prioritise consuming vegetables or salad first, followed by protein and fats, then carbohydrates. Eat slowly.
- Limit desserts.
- Ensure that reductions in calorie intake are small but consistent, around 200 kcal per day. Crash diets and dramatic drops don't work.
- Get adequate sleep, to keep your metabolism and hormones balanced.

You booze, you lose

As we age, we metabolise alcohol differently, and to be frank it has no performance benefit, other than making us talk a good game. In fact, it's long been known as a disruptor of sleep quantity and quality and therefore recovery. It compromises the immune system, decreases reaction time, impairs cognitive performance, reduces hormone secretion, blocks fat burning and slows recovery rate from injury.

A study showed that exercise followed by alcohol caused the signals that would normally tell your body to adapt and get stronger to be suppressed immediately. Another study calculated that booze negatively affects protein synthesis by 37%, a huge negative impact on our recovery from hard runs, strength workouts and injury.

Alcohol can also affect heart rhythms, even in low doses. As you may have seen from your parents at Christmas, our ability to tolerate alcohol worsens with age. **Two beers a day over a year, incidentally, shrinks your brain to the same extent as a decade of ageing.** Pint, anyone?

'How you feel about running is also how you feel about your whole life.'

TOM HUTCHISON

Tom, seventy-two, is a lifelong runner, a retired paediatrician and now heavily involved in local athletics. It wasn't until his fifties that he trained more consistently, and the work bore fruit with a marathon PB at fifty-five and four England masters vests in his sixties and seventies. Unusually, Tom has over fifteen years of certified VO_2 max data, which gives us an illuminating insight into his running physiology. In 2025 Tom ran a 3:31 marathon, the fourth-fastest time for a V70 in Britain that year.

My parents didn't run and they never encouraged me to, but a PE teacher did and I ran cross-country as a teenager. As an under-seventeen I represented Warwickshire at the National Schools in Blackburn. I was sixth team counter in eighteenth place and we won. As an adult, as I moved around the country, I would usually join running clubs and I got into trail running, too.

When I had three small kids, a friend would call round at 6.30 a.m. twice a week. We'd run together for an hour, chat about work and life. I moved to Bath and was running occasional marathons – I could run sub-three hours then – then stop training, start again. I've had every sort of injury at some point, but nothing that's kept me out for long.

I was approaching fifty, a bit overweight and I decided to do the New York Marathon. I trained quite hard for it and ran 3:20, which wasn't particularly good for me. But I'd lost some weight and I liked feeling fit. That was a turning point. My kids were older, more independent, so I had a bit more time. I joined Team Bath Athletic Club, went to Tuesday night track sessions, working up to maybe 40 miles a week.

That was my best spell of running, starting at fifty – and it was a midlife thing, if I'm honest. It was about body image, how you feel about yourself. I'm a fairly ordinary heterosexual male and I notice if someone likes me, if someone flirts with me. Younger people flirt all the time, but once you reach a certain age, you become invisible. You don't realise it's a thing, until it isn't any more. I lost my hair when I was around fifty too and it just hits your confidence. How you feel about running is also how you feel about your whole life. So I just wanted to feel good about myself physically and to keeping training well just suited me fine.

I wanted to get a Good For Age (GFA) time for the London Marathon and I ran 3:14 at the Lochaber Marathon aged fifty, which was enough, and I held a GFA time for years, doing a marathon somewhere every year until the Covid lockdown. As I worked at it, my time got better and better and I ran my marathon PB of 2:57 at fifty-five. Nowadays I tend to run 3:31–3:40.

I've been fortunate to represent my country as a masters runner via both British Masters and England Athletics. I've had an England vest for the marathon and at masters international cross-country meets, for V65 and V70 teams. In one of them I was really pleased to place second V65.

England won and there was a gala dinner afterwards.

Every time I get into a new age category, I get excited about it. It's great, because you're at the top of the tree again. That's where the speed stuff that we do at the club really helps. At the Tokyo Marathon, I was looking at runners and times beforehand and aiming to be the first V70. A local guy showed up and ran faster, but I was the fastest V70 European and that was just fine. I was more happy about the way I did it, being efficient, not wasting time.

I have VO_2 max and blood lactate data from ages fifty-six to seventy-two and it does show a performance decline, as one would expect. But encouragingly, the data shows very similar athletic performance between ages sixty-eight and seventy-two, with only fractionally higher heart rate for the same paces. In fact, my first lactate threshold is exactly the same as it was five years ago, and my running economy has increased slightly. My current VO_2 max of 48.4 is classified as 'excellent' for my age and is very similar to four years ago and the report says I can still improve on my current data. There's a clear arresting of decline from when I started doing regular strength work, around age fifty-eight.

Overall, though, running is getting harder and harder. There's fewer and fewer people – I just see people succumbing to cancer all around me. Also, the decline even amongst those training hard does seem significant. I have to be careful, because I got niggles this year from cross-country and the track. I knew what it was and I knew what I'd done. I just backed off for a while, and came back gradually. I thought, *You know what? I'm just not going to do 800-metre repeats for a while, because I don't need to.* You have to think more carefully about what you do.

My partner's very fit too, an elite-level sabre fencer, and we like that about each other. We've got friends where one person does a lot of sport and the partner does absolutely nothing and they find it quite hard to understand each other's needs. All of our three children are sporty, though we never pushed that. I went running – I was doing my own thing. But they've all become runners, too, some to a pretty high standard.

One year at Christmas, before they were serious about running but showing some interest, I bought all of them a pair of new running shoes and entered us all into a Boxing Day race. That was probably 1993 and we're still doing it almost every Christmas – it's became quite competitive! It's a social thing, involving the family. I select most of my races now around what friends and family are doing.

STRETCH GOALS

So, sleep and diet are the big ones. Both change as we age and need our attention. What else is worth doing to maximise performance and recovery and reduce our chances of getting niggles or worse?

Once we're in our fifties, warming up, which younger runners may have got away with ignoring (guilty!), becomes essential. Our muscles are tighter and connective tissues lose elasticity, a one–two punch that slows us down by shortening our stride and increasing injury risk. So expressing a full range of motion (ROM) should become a priority. A short bout of pre-run dynamic stretching improves ROM and reduces injury risk, found a 2021 study, and may even boost our VO2 max and running economy.[43]

'You can lose 10–15% of your range of motion and not even know it,' says Nicholas DiNubile. 'Runners commonly develop tightness in the calves, low back, hip flexors and hamstrings, which hinders your stretch/reflex response, literally removing spring from your step and slowing your pace.' Warm up, he advises, to aid flexibility (how far a muscle or joint can move) and mobility (how efficiently you can control that ROM). 'Get the blood and synovial fluids flowing [through connective tissues] to lubricate your joints.' A warm-up is especially important if we're planning to run with intensity.

Static stretches (held for up to 30 seconds) can inhibit performance if done pre-run, because they decrease the muscles' potential to store elastic energy and increase the risk of strain, but can be beneficial post-run. Instead, pre-run stretches should be dynamic. This means movements such as:

- bounding
- hopping
- jumping
- walking lunges
- side lunges
- leg swings
- walking single-leg deadlifts
- heel-to-bum kicks.

A warm-up should take 10–15 minutes, the amount of time it takes for our fascia – the springy connective tissue that encases our muscles – to loosen up. Strides, too, could be part of a warm-up routine, though ease into them. If these are alien ideas, consider joining a local running club on a track or workout/intervals night and the coach should lead you through a dynamic warm-up routine.

Static post-run stretching helps to promote blood flow to the muscles, which enables them to repair and recover more quickly, remove waste products, and reduce any muscle and joint soreness. This can improve the flexibility of ROM, leaving you less susceptible to strains and overuse injuries. Post-run stretches could include:

- hamstring stretch
- glute stretch
- groin stretch
- calf stretch
- soleus (lower calf) stretch
- hip flexor stretch
- quadriceps stretch
- back/upper-body stretch (such as downward dog).

If a combination of pre- and post-run stretching and strength work leaves you feeling like you still lack flexibility and mobility, see a physiotherapist or try this mobility and activation session from Team Bath Athletic Club: **teambathac.org/training-resources-videos**

Don't shoot the massager

We're bombarded with recovery ideas, even more so if there's a related gadget to be sold. How many are worth our money and time? Compared to their popular usage among amateur and elite runners, the scientifically proven benefits of foam rollers, percussive tools and even massages are surprisingly scant and mixed.

Massage reduces DOMS (delayed-onset muscle soreness), perceived fatigue and improves flexibility (though that may be less beneficial for running economy), but is expensive and time-consuming, carries some risk and no positive effects have been proven for performance. Yet elite runners swear by it and coaches recommend it (I too feel like there's an injury-prevention benefit in releasing tight muscles and tendons).

Massage guns used immediately post-workout *may* reduce DOMS and improve performance after an exhaustive workout, say studies. Foam rolling after intense workouts can relieve soreness over the next two days, according to a 2014 study, and *may* increase flexibility and ROM. But another study suggested it has more benefit as a warm-up activity.

Compression garments, namely socks, worn during recovery have been shown to decrease muscle soreness, and subsequent performance has improved. Inflatable 'legs' help with deep-vein thrombosis symptoms, as do compression socks, but there's limited research on athletes.

Active recovery, including light jogging, aqua exercise and yoga, may help to reduce DOMS when done within 24–48 hours after an intense workout. Passive recovery – in other words inactivity or total rest – is commonly thought to be great for recovery. The older the athlete, the more passive recovery is likely to be the best option, says Joe Friel.

Yoga is popular with runners, but its benefit for performance is largely unproven. Yoga is essentially concentrated stretching or lengthening of our muscles, and we know that static stretching before running reduces our economy by 3–7%. A 2017 study found that dynamic stretching improved performance slightly, with no change in injury rates. Distance runners who are less flexible tend to be more economical, found another study, so inflexible runners may be better athletes. Indeed, another study showed that shouting motivational phrases improved performance more than yoga did. So, the jury is still out on yoga for mature runners. But if you feel it works for you, keep downward dogging, ideally after consulting an in-person physiotherapist.

Ice baths and cold-water immersion have become popular but have been shown to slow, reduce or even stop the body's natural healing process, preventing blood flow to the damaged tissues and slowing transportation of the by-products of inflammation. Cold-water immersion negatively impacts adaptations from strength training, with as much as two-thirds less muscle mass gained, found a 12-week study.

Evidence of saunas and other heat protocols *as recovery methods* is also sparse, though a 2016 study showed hot baths increase circulation to fatigued muscles and joints.[44] But they do have training, mental health and longevity benefits.

We know that heat training increases plasma and blood volume, which brings positive fitness and health adaptations, including heart health, blood pressure, vascular function, respiratory health, cerebral blood flow, mental well-being/happiness, cognitive health, better sleep and performance, and longevity. Sauna exposure also releases that precious human growth hormone, raising it by as much as 150%.

An eight-week study in sauna use saw a 9% increase in VO2 max, albeit in sedentary adults. Thirty minutes in a sauna immediately after training for three weeks resulted in an improvement in the time to exhaustion on a treadmill run by 32%, in competitive male distance runners and triathletes.[45] A twenty-year study of 2,300 Finnish men found a reduced mortality risk of 40% with usage four to seven times per week, along with a 50% lower cardiovascular risk, 66% lower dementia risk and 65% lower Alzheimer's risk.[46] A study of 524 Finnish octogenarians reported that physical function, vitality, social functioning and general health were considerably better in sauna users than in non-users.[47] Ideal protocols are debated, but something like 15–20 minutes every other day should bring significant health and performance benefits.[48]

While some studies have shown benefits from cupping, ranging from improvements in blood cholesterol levels to pain relief, most peer-reviewed science is not as supportive of the technique. Similarly, with the ancient art of acupuncture, the Mayo Clinic points out 'there's also evidence that acupuncture works best in people who expect it to work', which links neatly to the placebo effect.

Placebos are things we gain a tangible benefit from merely by believing they work, and have been shown to improve symptoms of everything from coughs and pain to depression and even Parkinson's disease. In one study, competitive cyclists were informed that they would be given a zero, low or high dose of caffeine before a time trial, but all of them were actually given a placebo. Over the 10-kilometre race, athletes who thought they had received a low dose performed 1.5% better than baseline, while those expecting a high dose performed 3% better.[49]

A big part of rest and recovery is mental, so if we do something we enjoy – whether that's foam rolling or bingeing on Netflix – it's probably going to make us feel at our best. If a runner thinks they're doing something that will boost their ability or recovery, they may relax or sleep better, and that might be enough.

Talking of placebos, the expectation effect shows that our beliefs can be more powerful than our DNA. One of my favourite studies involved some runners being told they had a 'special gene' for performance, while the other group was told they lacked it.[50] Those told they had the magical gene consequently ran faster, recovered quicker and outperformed the other athletes. Because they believed they could. Meanwhile, runners in the other group collapsed under their false beliefs, fatiguing early. They thought they were weak. But many in the latter cohort did have a rare genetic trait that helps clear carbon dioxide and use oxygen more efficiently. On paper they were better athletes. **Those who outperformed did so simply because they believed they could.** Their heart rate data improved, their lactate threshold improved, they processed oxygen like elite runners. **The mind literally changed the body. Now what if we all started believing we were biologically ten years younger than we chronologically are?** After all, we could be.

What else can the mature athlete do towards optimal ageing and performance? Sometimes it's about removing lifestyle elements that are working against us. In ultramarathons, we say 'beware the chair' about checkpoints, but this translates to everyday life, too. There's a good case for cutting down on sitting time (standing desk for the win!), although this will have greater impact on the sedentary. The enzymes that help us fight fat drop by 50% when we spend the day sitting. That fat stays in our bloodstream, circulating and piling up in our blood vessels. Watching TV for four or more hours a day increases our risk of dying from heart disease by 80% compared to watching for just two hours.[51] A study of 800,000 people found those who sat the most had a twofold increase in diabetes, a twofold increase in cardiovascular disease risk and a 50% increased risk of early death. Rest is good, but not that type. That doesn't apply wholesale to us runners, unless perhaps the only time we're not sitting is during a run. Consider exercise snacks. A study showed that both 3-minute squat breaks and 3-minute walking breaks every 45 minutes led to much healthier blood sugar patterns compared to sitting all day.[52]

Toxic plasticity

From a health perspective, another big issue is trying to minimise microplastics, nanoplastics and forever chemicals. We are consuming hundreds to thousands of plastic particles every day, through our soil, sewage sludge, grass, toilet paper, food, milk, air and water. These microplastics usually go hand in hand with forever chemicals, which as the name suggests are toxic and last a very long time. Their horrifying omnipresence and the scope of their effects are only likely to grow, thinks American biomedical scientist Dr Rhonda Patrick.

Forever chemicals or microplastics are found in plastic bottles, food packaging (including pizza boxes), non-stick pans, cooking utensils, beauty products, hygiene products, cleaning products, clothing, bedding, candles, teabags and even 'paper' receipts. Shellfish are highly contaminated. They're also found in our blood, brain, heart, liver, lungs, breast milk and semen – in 100% of samples taken from humans and dogs. Microplastics are accumulating in our brain at ten times the rate of other organs. 'That's incredibly disturbing,' says Patrick, who believes the chemicals increase neuroinflammation and much of that comes mostly from the air, with a higher risk in polluted urban areas.

People living near golf courses have a 126% higher risk of Parkinson's disease compared to people living six miles away, probably due to pesticides and herbicides transferred in ground water.[53] Firefighting foam, often found at airports, is especially potent with forever chemicals. A third of British waterways which provide drinking water have unacceptably high levels of forever chemicals. Another study found forever chemical trifluoroacetic acid (TFA) in thirty-one of thirty-two British rivers sampled.[54] '[It's] everywhere,' a researcher told the BBC. 'We will all be drinking water containing TFA every day – so we'll be exposed throughout our lifetime. It's that long-term, low-level exposure that is the big concern.'

The exact effects on us are yet to be fully understood, but we know BPAs, BPSs, PFAs, phthalates (often disguised as 'fragrance' or 'perfume') and other forever chemicals are endocrine disruptors. They mimic oestrogen and disrupt our hormones, and this is linked to increased blood pressure, type 2 diabetes, cardiovascular disease and cancer, and can also affect children's development, including links to autism and ADHD. Post-mortem analysis of people with dementia found ten times more micro-plastic particles in their brain. Forever chemicals are linked to cancer, liver damage, immune function and fertility issues, causing hypospadias and undescended testicles.

From a runner's perspective, there are implications for our metabolism. Microplastics 'cause noticeable structural changes, such as swelling and a loss of integrity in the mitochondria, reducing ATP synthesis'.[55] BPA also affects calcium signalling, a kind of switch or language spoken between our hormones, nerves, genes and muscles, crucial in regulating a wide range of vital cellular processes. It's a very minimal win to know that we runners may sweat out some BPAs, but that'll be a tiny percentage of what's going into us. Patrick advises that we:

- avoid heating food in plastic (heat rapidly accelerates leaching of chemicals)
- avoid hot drinks in plastic-lined takeaway cups
- avoid food in black plastic containers, which could include known carcinogens
- avoid drinking from plastic bottles – canned food, canned drinks

and glass bottles can also have toxic chemicals in their plastic lining and lids
- consider high-quality water filters (reverse osmosis filters – though they remove good minerals too) and air filters for our home
- eat broccoli, sprouts and cabbage, which all include sulforaphane, which can help detoxify us from BPA.

She also advises that dietary fibre may help prevent absorption by helping the chemicals move through us quickly.

'It's a mind thing, isn't it? Don't let the old man in.'

GUY WOODS

Guy, sixty-three, a Bath-based landscape gardener, was British Masters V55 Champion at 5K and 10K, and has represented GB at the World Masters Cross-Country championships and World Masters Mountain Running Championships, winning team gold in both. Despite injury setbacks and operations, Guy continues to train hard but innovatively. He also beat this author, fourteen years his junior, in a sprint finish to win Wiltshire's popular Slaughterford 9 multi-terrain race.

I love multi-terrain races, cross-country and short fell races, and to get fit for those I would do lots of 5Ks and 10Ks (my 5K PB is 14:50, my 10K PB is 31:50). When the kids had grown up and left, suddenly I had this window and if you haven't got any other major hobbies, you can get really fit, fit enough to get an international vest. That was my main goal: get selected and hopefully have a good run. Which I did.

I do get more niggles now and my job doesn't help there. Landscape gardening is tough on the knees. When I was fifty, I had a knee operation and the surgeon said, 'You shouldn't be running every day – you've got to do more cross-training.' I took his word for it and bought an elliptical machine.

It's bloody brilliant. It means I can go harder in my sessions and I recover a lot better. I don't think I went backwards at all, in fact I was still progressing in my age group. I do HIIT sessions, 8 x 1 minute with 30-second recoveries, you know, bang, bang, bang. I came back and placed second in my first race. So I really did bounce back from that operation. The other great machine I've got is a Nordic cross-country machine.

When running, my classic workout is 12 x 400 metres in about 75–77 seconds with 200 metres jog recovery. I always do one hill workout a week, my graveyard session, 10 repetitions of 200 metres uphill. And at least once in a month, I do a longer hill session on a 3-minute hill, 8 repetitions. For quite a few years, I've done almost exactly the same sessions. I train in the red zone and the green zone, not in the grey zone. So my easy runs are really easy (although they are hilly). But all the other stuff is right in the red zone, especially the hill reps, literally being sick at the top of the hill. I was also doing parkruns once a fortnight.

Twice a month I do a weighted walk, around 30K and 1,200 metres of ascent, carrying 7 kilograms. I Nordic pole as well. I love my walking. I walked the Galician Way recently, I've done the Alta Via 1 in the Dolomites, I'm planning to go across the Pyrenees. These aren't competitive at all. They're just adventures. Being on your feet for a length of time is great training. But as we get into these older brackets, I suppose we have to be a bit more careful, a bit more selective with what we're doing.

I do loads of strength work. Pull-ups, chin-ups, I was averaging 300 press-ups a day. I would just drop down and bang out 50 at a time. Romanian deadlifts, Nordic curls – I made my own Nordic machine out of scaffold, my wife thought I was having a heart attack. I use a 30-degree slant board and do all my squats on that. That's transformed the strength in my knees. It's not strength training for hours and hours a day. It's easy to fit all this stuff in. I'm always doing some form of exercise: hip flexor exercises while watching the TV, a few yoga moves. I like hanging as well. I hang from a bar for two minutes every day. I do quite a bit of plyometrics. The classic 30-second calf raises as you clean your teeth. Once you get it into your head, there's a little routine, people don't even notice, you just sneak off and do something. I do enjoy it. It's not a chore for me. I find it difficult to sit still.

For recovery, I swim every day, about a mile, takes me about 30 minutes; then I do 15 minutes of aqua jogging, in the flow lane with the old ladies, purely for recovery. I think it's fantastic.

I was vegetarian for twenty years, but about fifteen years ago I introduced meat back into my diet, because I do love the taste, so I eat it twice a week. But I eat mostly wholefoods, I'm just making a pistou soup now. My wife's into nutrition as well. We're into kefirs, stuff like that, for gut health. I've had no alcohol for fifteen years, apart from occasional wedding toasts. It never really agreed with me. I'm in bed by 9.30, though I'm an early bird and cannot sleep past 5 in the morning.

Anyway, that's the training and the lifestyle that got me to be 5K and 10K British Masters Champion at V55. And run a 16:20 parkrun aged fifty-seven.

I did initially struggle with the idea I'm ageing. Especially on Strava, you can get a bit green-eyed – 'Oh God, I could have run that in my sleep' and all that. I have struggled. But I've embraced it now. The age-graded stuff is genius. You can look at it and see you've still managed a 92% age grade for that time, you know, even though you came 900th. That keeps you mentally competitive.

I mean, I'll go to every race still trying to win it, right? But obviously that's not going to happen any more. So the second one down is my age category, the third one is age-graded time. I'll always try and win my age category, or try and beat as many thirty-year-olds as I can!

It's a mind thing, isn't it? Don't let the old man in.

YOUNG MINDS RUN FREE

When I delved into all this ageing lark, the biggest surprise to me was that the way we think can significantly affect our biological ageing. It sounds fanciful, but **it's scientifically proven that we can literally think ourselves younger**. Positive expectations about ageing lead to a longer, healthier life, while negative beliefs can be hugely detrimental, according to several robust studies spanning five decades.[56]

In a landmark 1979 Harvard University experiment, a group of seventy- to eighty-year-olds were placed in a week-long retreat at a location in the style of the late 1950s and were strongly encouraged to live as if it was that decade.[57] Everything, from the décor to the films and music, was from that period. They had to talk about 1950s political and sporting events as if they were currently in progress, and write a biography of themselves for that era in the present tense. The researchers also ran a second retreat where, while most factors remained the same, they were asked to reminisce about the past without acting as if they were reliving that period.

Most participants showed improvements from baseline tests, but the first group saw the greatest benefits: 63% made significant gains in the cognitive tests, compared to 44% in the control group. In addition, their vision, hearing, posture and dexterity improved, their joints were more flexible and their inflammation from arthritis had receded.

A Yale study asked 660 people with an average age of sixty-three to rate their level of agreement with the statement 'as you get older, you are less useful'.[58] Researchers found the average person with a more positive attitude lived for 22.6 years post-study, while the average person with poorer interpretations of ageing survived for just 15 years.

Other studies have concluded that **many people will endorse negative ageist beliefs long before they start experiencing age-related disability themselves.** And those views, expressed in people's mid-thirties, can predict their subsequent risk of cardiovascular disease up to thirty-eight years later.

Age beliefs may play a key role in the development of Alzheimer's disease, another study found. Tracking 4,765 participants over four years, researchers discovered that positive expectations of ageing halved the risk of developing the disease, compared to those who saw old age as an inevitable period of decline.[59] (This was even true of people who carried a harmful variant of the APOE gene that renders people more susceptible to the disease.) A positive mindset can counteract an inherited misfortune, protecting against the build-up of the toxic plaques and neuron loss that characterise Alzheimer's.

Merely feeling old makes the brain age faster. In a study, adults who perceived themselves as older showed greater loss of grey matter in key brain regions, independent of their real chronological age. Indeed, elderly people who have been primed with negative age stereotypes tend to have higher systolic blood pressure in response to challenges, while those who have seen positive stereotypes demonstrate a more muted reaction.[60] Essentially, if we believe we are frail and helpless, small difficulties start to feel more threatening. Over the long term, this heightened stress response increases levels of bodily inflammation and cortisol, which could both raise the risk of ill health.

In people with negative age beliefs, telomere dysfunction is accelerated and their cells look biologically older. In those with positive attitudes, it's much slower and their cells appear younger. If we associate age with frailty and disability, we may be less likely to exercise as we get older and that lack of activity is going to increase our predisposition to illnesses. It's remarkable stuff when you think about it. As well as getting us out of the door on that dark and wet January morning, our mindset may add several years to our life. The way we think about ageing shapes the way we age. If we think we're slowing down and becoming less of an athlete, we will be. If we think we can still be an ageless ace, we can be.

'The greatest obstacle to better performance is psychological, not physiological,' says Joe Friel in *Fast After 50*. 'Your head needs to say yes. Most people simply lack the motivation to do what it takes.' He adds: 'You aren't old until age becomes your excuse.'

Acceptance and possibility

Will that be enough, though, when we see our parkrun times slowing? There's a lot more we midlife runners can do to get the most out of our running. 'My approach is acceptance,' says Dr Josephine Perry, sports psychologist, runner and author of *The Ten Pillars of Success*. Acceptance and Commitment Therapy is about trying to notice unhelpful thoughts we're having and learning to sit alongside them rather than fight them. 'I'm not as fast as I used to be.' 'That person looks younger than me.' 'Why is my pace so slow?'

People can advocate better for themselves, Perry says. 'It might be, "I'm not twenty-five any more, but I do own a house, I do have a child and I've got a much better-paying job." So we should look at balancing out those things.' Instead of unhelpful thoughts, Perry says, '**Let's see what's possible at this stage of life**.' Runners can shape the narrative in their head around that. And age has advantages, as we'll see.

'Embrace it,' adds Perry, whose co-host on the *Be Braver* podcast is Annie Emerson, a former professional triathlete who ran a 2:52 marathon in her fifties. The image on their podcast socials is Emerson doing a handstand. 'I see quite a lot on Instagram, too: "I'm trying to get a sub-three-hour marathon in my fifties."'

Perry also cites her Sunday gymnastics class as a moment of **embracing both age and silliness**. 'Most of us are women in our forties with kids and it's our 90 minutes of being childish. Nobody is there pretending they're thirty. We are embracing the fact that we're doing something really silly, fun and cool in our late forties.'

At the risk of a horrible name drop, I was once hanging out in a camp ground in Frozen Head State Park, Tennessee, listening to two runners talking about ageing. They were both beyond fifty and they spoke about how they were slowing down physically, but also about their remaining, impressively ambitious, running goals. One was Ireland's multi-record-breaking athlete and three-time Winter Spine Race winner Eoin Keith (more on page 91); the other was Gary Cantrell, aka Lazarus Lake, creator of the Barkley Marathons and the backyard ultra concept, and a lifelong ultrarunner. 'I often remind myself that I'll never be as fast as I am today,' concluded Eoin. And that really stuck with me – the acceptance, truth and curiosity of it.

Age grouping/grading is another really effective way to stay mentally and physically engaged with running. After all, it just makes running fairer. For most of our lives we only compete against those of a similar age to us. Even as thirty-year-olds, we weren't competing with fifteen-year-olds or sixty-five-year-olds. Indeed, it's probably only truly between the ages of around twenty to forty – just 25% or less of our life – when we don't really think about our age category. Age grading is a wonderful equaliser which excites midlife running friends of mine.

Parkrun junkies know all about age-graded percentage, and indeed this is often all they seem to care about. 'Age grading seeks to "level the playing field",' explains the parkrun website. Take, for example, these four parkrunners: a nine-year-old girl who runs 29:15, a twenty-three-year-old male who runs 21:30, a sixty-five-year-old man with 27:57, and a seventy-five-year-old woman with 40:25. Who's fastest? Although their times are different, they all share exactly the same age-graded percentage score of 60% when age and sex are taken into account.

Sixty per cent is fairly speedy. The score is the ratio of your own finish time against the world record for your sex and age, expressed as a percentage. If you take forty minutes to complete a parkrun and the world record for your age and sex is twenty minutes, your age-graded percentage score is 50%. On top of that, parkrun throws in data for each specific course.

Parkrun's algorithm is based on World Masters Athletics (WMA) data. Every few years, WMA statisticians review global race records to identify the best possible time an athlete can run distances from 5K to the marathon. Then they use a formula to calculate an age factor for every age, which serves as the 'best possible time' an athlete of that gender and age should be able to run, to compare times with athletes from all over the world.

A seventy-year-old woman might run a half marathon and place 223rd, while a thirty-year-old man finishes 35th. Yet that thirty-year-old achieved an age-grade score of 70% against thirty-year-old males globally, whereas the female athlete ran a time very close to the top time expected for a seventy-year-old woman, registering a 91% grade score and a superior performance. And suddenly the world is fairer.

Age grading allows thrilling inter-family feuds – is your seventeen-year-old son *really* faster than you? – and you can even compare yourself, with biological fairness, to your younger self. Are you closer to optimal fitness now as a sixty-year-old than when you were twenty-five? You may never match that 10K PB from fifteen years ago, but you can aspire to achieve the same 10K age grade score for your current age. You might discover that, although slower in absolute terms, your current times are of relatively higher quality. Or you could aim to run a regional, national or even world-class 5K time. Suddenly, approaching that fiftieth or sixtieth birthday with the heady idea of being one of the youngest in a new category has some excitement attached. Just search 'age-grading calculator' online or check out the excellent *Skamper* app.

Age grading definitely helps mature athletes, says Perry. 'A lot of athletes I work with will set age-grading goals, or age-graded goals, so you can still feel like you're moving forward. I like the idea of setting PBs for certain stages in our lives, the most obvious one being for women coming back from having a baby. I know my 5K PB from when I was twenty-nine, but I also know my post-baby PB. That felt like such a fundamental shift in my life and my body that it felt very fair to allow myself to reset. I suggest that for lots of women who might be struggling with "My body's changed". You can do that for a post-menopausal PB or a post-fifty PB, too.'

Values and purpose

Being fully aware of our values is another way to stay engaged with our running. 'Your values tend to change a bit as you get older,' says Perry. 'I never had the value of family before I had my daughter, but now that's really important to me and I want to role-model hard work and effort. So I use that in my running: that I'm not slowing down, because I want Hattie to be proud of me as a mummy. If I've whipped out and not got that medal, how can I look her in the face and how can I teach her the things I want to teach her? Your values might change, but you can use your values very powerfully.' Perry encourages runners to think about their values and not just leave them as a vague idea. She recommends deciding on a minimum of three and trying to live our life – and do our running – in accordance with them. That way, we'll feel more fulfilled.

Related to values, a sense of purpose is a very powerful tool, too. The runners she's worked with who struggle the most are those who have a purpose that's about themselves. 'When somebody is purely focused on "me", it is harder to get the best out of yourself because you've got no wider purpose.' On the other hand, take someone like Eddie Brocklesby, 'A mad old woman still doing Ironman at age 81!', according to her Instagram bio. She's eighty-two now and when she was in her mid-seventies, she was doing an Ironman and her saddle broke on her bike mid-race. 'For most of us, we'd be like, "Excellent. I can quit now," because this is a really good excuse. But her purpose is to spread the message that we need to stay active in retirement.'

Eddie runs a charity called SilverFit that keeps retirees active and social. 'They meet up, they have a cup of tea. They do walking, football, netball or badminton, they have another cup of tea, and they go home. They spend three hours with friends, being active. That's her passion. It is really important for her that she finishes the Ironman, so she has a platform on which to talk about her charity. If a seventy-five-year-old woman finishes an Ironman, people want to talk to her, so she gets that opportunity to talk about the importance of being active while you age. So she had to finish that Ironman to do it, so instead of using it as a really good excuse to quit, she stood up, cycled standing up for the next 40 kilometres and then ran the marathon, because it meant she would still cross the finish line and be able to talk about what really mattered to her.'

Perry urges runners to draw a Venn diagram (three circles that overlap in the middle) and think about what they're really good at, what they love and what makes them angry when they watch the news or scroll Instagram.

For Perry, that led to encouraging equal coverage of female and male sport as her purpose.

She advises us to also – at all ages – concentrate on process or input goals. Output goals might be a race time or placing, while input goals are what you want to input into your race. 'That might be about behaviour, it might be about a task, an action. What inputs are you putting into your run? You're not in control of your output, but you're totally in control of your input.' An input might be to concentrate on good technique, to fuel or hydrate well, or to smile more.

'If you focus on the outputs, it triggers your threat system and you end up not being able to run very well. If you focus on inputs, you're entirely in control, it makes you feel much better. There's no threat system triggered, so you're much more relaxed and you can run faster. You're not measuring your self-worth and what those outcomes are, which you've got no control over whatsoever. You'll probably get better outcomes and better outputs, because you are focused on the right things.'

When we're younger, some of our inputs might be about the competitiveness of a race. 'Eilish McColgan's input goal or mantra is "stay", because she always goes out as fast as she can and then hangs on for dear life. I worked with someone whose only goal for a race was to be in discomfort. They wanted to put themselves in discomfort for 10K. They got a PB.'

We can adapt it to our age. 'It's always about what you might input. The beautiful thing is you can attach your inputs to your strengths and weaknesses. The athlete who got the PB realised she had great strength on the hills. It might be one of your inputs to hammer up the hills. And you can do that if you're sixteen or sixty-five.'

Perry suggests we give our input a score out of ten. 'Your eight out of ten for effort is going to be different on a day when you're doing 55K and it's 33 °C, than on a day where you're doing a half marathon in 12 °C, you're really fresh and you've had a great week at work. So your output will be different, but your effort level can be the same, because your brain is telling you, "This feels like eight out of ten that I've got in me right now." So you stop beating yourself up for outcomes you can't control.' That works at any stage of life.

Passion project

Passion is a word with a lot of power. I've always loved a story from Matt Fitzgerald's *How Bad Do You Want It? Mastering The Psychology of Mind Over Muscle,* where Ned Overend wins an XTERRA World Championship off-road triathlon aged forty-three. He was more than five years older than anyone to ever win a world championship in any major endurance sport, says Fitzgerald. How? Lots of training – in this case with variety and balance – and smart execution, sure. 'I don't mind training hard,' he told Fitzgerald, 'but I don't tend to do a lot of long training. I get out there and I don't dick around.' Ned never trained beyond his level of enthusiasm. Partly because of that, he still had passion.

Indeed those with positive attitudes and who don't sweat the small stuff tend to age slower and live longer, according to 1973 research entitled 'Longevity and the Longevity Syndrome'.[61] Scientists observing men and women aged 87–103 noted some common personality traits, including a tendency to '**see life as a great adventure**', 'optimism and a sense of humour' and 'freedom from anxiety'. More contemporary psychologists agree that similar traits are strongly predictive of longevity: **openness, conscientiousness, extraversion and low neuroticism**. Psychologists are still trying to work out why it's these characteristics, but the similarities among mature athletes excelling is uncanny, says Fitzgerald. A more neurotic-minded person will spend more time in stressful states, creating more cortisol, which is linked to weight gain and atrophy, with increased risk of Alzheimer's and other diseases. Conscientious people are less likely to drink; extroverted people are more likely to exercise. Fitzgerald links openness to coping styles. 'What we see in all of these men and women is limitless passion for sport and for the athletic lifestyle.' As a case in point, he cites the ever-smiley Haile Gebrselassie, who was still winning elite races aged thirty-nine and setting age-group world records in his forties.

'The wisdom of going where the joy and happiness leads is undeniable,' concludes Fitzgerald. 'If your passion endures, so will you.'

Mastery also gives us great hope. In *Mastery: The Keys to Success and Long-Term Fulfilment,* author George Leonard's view is that **mastery isn't an end goal. Instead, it's a path.** So it's about the journey and not the destination, the process and not the outcome. Mastery, says Leonard, is a lifelong journey of continuous learning, discovery and development of a skill, such as painting, teaching, chess, martial arts and, yes, running. He argues that modern culture teaches us to want the quick, easy and effortless way to success and happiness but never really gets us there. Instead, the master's path is the only sure-fire way to live a fulfilling life.

It's not too late. Gwendolyn Bounds is a great example of this. Her book *Not Too Late: The Power of Pushing Limits at Any Age* is about the power of working to get good at something new and hard whatever your age. She had an unexpected five-year path of transformation from an unathletic forty-five-year-old office executive glued to her screens into an age-group medallist and world championship competitor in obstacle course racing. But the key concept is that mastery is a *path,* rather than a goal. After all, we can never complete running, can we?

Ageless athletes should also ask themselves the biggest question of all: why do you run? 'For me, it's been to stay fit enough to have a good spine,' says Perry. 'But that's not very exciting and isn't the thing that usually gets me out of the door. I was really reflecting on this and then I went for a run up to Glastonbury Tor and I was like, "Oh, maybe this is my why", because through running I get to adventure, I get to see really cool things I wouldn't get to see otherwise, and you get to explore more of anywhere you go to, on your feet. That explains why I run. For other people, it might be about the social side, so doing marathon training on their own is just going to make them miserable and demotivated. But if they do the Monday track session, they do the Wednesday club run and they do a Sunday run with a friend, that's going to keep them in for longer. So, the more runners know why they run, the more they can max out on those reasons, and then they will stick with it for a lot longer.'

So, why do you run?

Ageless aces

We can still be the most kick-ass athlete we can be. Look at Nicky Spinks, Ludovic Pommeret, Eoin Keith and Jo Pavey. Think Tina Turner, Serena Williams, Harrison Ford returning as Indiana Jones (and as Han Solo for that matter), Sylvester Stallone as Rocky Balboa.

In the wider world, it's easy to assume most of the greatest things are achieved by irritatingly precocious twenty-three-year-olds called December or Silver. But think of Yuichiro Miura climbing Mount Everest aged eighty, Julia Child hosting her TV show into her eighties, Roger Robinson winning a masters cross-country championship at eighty-three, Mahatma Gandhi leading the Salt March to Dandi at sixty-one, Nelson Mandela becoming president of South Africa aged seventy-five and, er, Susan Boyle shooting to fame at the age of forty-eight.

These ageless aces aren't applying for their bus passes. They're planning on skidding into their graves sideways shouting 'Holy shit, what a ride!' … though not for a long time yet. They're sticking a defiant finger up at time. They're showing the A-word is just a number and they don't give a hoot what that number is. We can be like them. And a lot of that is to do with our attitude.

Talking of numbers, I very much liked a social media meme I saw recently which suggested we simply switch the word 'age' for 'level'. 'I'm at level 55' sounds a whole lot better and gives our number the status it deserves.

I may be biased towards the longer stuff, but it makes a shedload of sense to me that as we mature and know we won't get faster, maybe it's time to think about going longer. We can maybe be more competitive than we thought, but it's not really about that. It's hugely rewarding to stretch to a new distance, perhaps one we previously thought wasn't possible, such as 100K or 100 miles or even further. As I wrote this chapter, an eighty-year-old American man completed the notoriously hot, 135-mile Badwater ultramarathon. Now there's a guy defying his chronological age.

GOING LONGEVITY

'I am the healthiest person on the planet,' says millionaire Bryan Johnson. 'I am fitter than most teenagers. My skin is smoother than that of women in their twenties. I have more stamina in bed than men in their twenties [...] My mental health is at its peak.'

The Holy Grail of eternal youth or immortality has been an elusive prize sought throughout known history, by Christians, Arthurians and Adolf Hitler (as well as Indiana Jones). Longevity – or anti-ageing as it's more commonly called when targeting woman – has become an arms race.

In September 2025, Russian president Vladimir Putin was overheard discussing immortality with Chinese president Xi Jinping. Putin suggested eternal life could be achievable as human organs can be continuously transplanted. 'In the past, it used to be rare for someone to be older than seventy, and these days they say that at seventy, one's still a child. People can live younger and younger, and even achieve immortality.'

'There's a chance of someone living to 150 this century,' Xi replied, via his translator.

Bryan Johnson is on a similar mission, minus all the invading and empire-building. Each morning, the American wakes at 4.30 a.m., takes a concoction of pills and supplements (around 40, but it used to be around 100), exercises, eats his last 'meal' (a carefully concocted smoothie) at 11 a.m. and is in bed again for 8.30 p.m., going through a routine of longevity protocols that cost him $2m a year. Johnson, star of Netflix documentary *Don't Die: The Man Who Wants to Live Forever,* claims his cardiovascular capacity is equal to the top 1% of eighteen-year-olds, his levels of body inflammation are 85% below the average eighteen-year-old and he is now ageing at a slower pace than 99% of twenty-year-olds. He's determined not to die. He's vegan and alcohol-free, has had blood transfusions from his seventeen-year-old son, measures his night-time erections and shares all of this on social media.

The phrase 'killing yourself to stay alive' springs to mind again, but he's a fascinating character and controversial pin-up star of the burgeoning and often weird longevity industry, trying to make us – or at least them – endure as long as possible. His actions may get people thinking about how much we can do, want to do, or indeed *should* do to enhance our longevity.

All sorts of biohacking research is ongoing, manipulating the age of cells and extending the lives of an increasing range of animals. Old mice eyes have been reprogrammed, for example, with them regaining sight. Young blood can rejuvenate old blood, it's thought, and a growing industry is keen on ideas such as reprogramming our bodies with gene therapy and resetting our cellular system. It feels weird, elitist and perhaps vain, but the topics of healthspan and longevity aren't growing old any time soon. The good news is that we midlife maestro runners are doing almost all of the key things already.

Into the Blue Zones

Understandably, there's a great deal of interest in Blue Zones, where people live longest, suffer less disease and enjoy better mental health and happiness. There are examples in Japan, Greece, Italy, Costa Rica and California. What we know is that their residents tend to eat more fruit, vegetables and whole foods, and less meat than westernised countries. It's thought that they don't overeat, only consume moderate amounts of alcohol, exercise regularly, and tend to have less stress and more purpose.

Purpose is rarely an individual pursuit in the Blue Zones. 'It's usually social, rooted in service, to family, to community, to something greater, philanthropic,' says Dan Buettner, author of *The Blue Zones: Secrets for Living Longer* and producer of Netflix's *Live to 100*, who says only 30% of us have purpose in our work. 'True purpose is found where your values, passions and strengths intersect. Where you can use them to give back.'

In Blue Zones, people tend to have wider family networks living close by or together. Indeed, loneliness is a silent killer (over half the adults in the US say they feel lonely). From a health perspective, loneliness is equivalent to smoking fifteen cigarettes a day. Having good and loving relationships and social bonds physically alters our DNA and adds eight years to our life, whereas not having such relationships doubles our chances of dying from any cause. 'Your friends shape your future more than you think,' says Buettner. 'If your closest friends are unhealthy, unhappy or isolated, those behaviours rub off, they're measurably contagious – you're 150% more likely to adopt those behaviours too, including unhappiness and even loneliness.' But joy, movement and deep connection are contagious, too. 'Surround yourself with people who challenge you, move with you [literally for runners], have meaningful conversations and show up on your worst days.'

Indeed, having close relationships is the biggest predictor of long-term well-being, according to the Harvard Study of Adult Development.[62] The study, conducted over eighty-five years, tracked people from their teens to their nineties, and found that the quality of relationships at fifty predicted health at eighty better than cholesterol, blood pressure or genes. High-quality relationships protect our bodies from chronic inflammation and improve immune health.

Another study predicted a good marriage can literally add years to your life, 7–9 for men and 2–4 for women.[63] 'Build that partnership, communicate and never keep score,' says Buettner. 'A strong relationship is a very powerful longevity tool.'

'It's not how many followers you have [on social media],' says performance coach Steve Magness, 'but who would answer the phone at 2 a.m.'

'I wish I had stayed in touch with my friends' and 'I wish that I had let myself be happier' were two key observations in the bestselling *The Top Five Regrets of the Dying*, by palliative care nurse Bronnie Ware. The other three were, 'I wish I hadn't worked so hard', 'I wish I'd had the courage to express my feelings' and 'I wish I'd had the courage to live a life true to myself, not the life others expected of me'. The last of these is the most common regret of all. 'Health brings a freedom very few realise, until they no longer have it,' wrote Ware.

Volunteering is also one of the most effective things we can do for mental health and longevity. With the 'helper's high' shown to lower stress and boost self-confidence and life satisfaction, we can make new friends and learn new skills. It gives us purpose, even decreases chronic pain, and those who volunteer live longer than those who don't.[64] So get cutting up the bananas at your local race's aid station.

Learning a new skill after forty decreases dementia risk by 40% and may also help slow time. Indeed, time feels faster as we age because our brains tend to record fewer new experiences. Novelty slows time. Routine speeds it up.

In summary

The first lesson is: don't stop. Ever. We're swimming upstream, so any time our arms don't plunge into the water ahead of us, we get pushed a little further down the ageing river and we may not be able to get back to that point. Consistency is key, though that means being flexible, being deliberate with recovery and seeing a physio sooner rather than later, now we know what's at stake. We also need to keep an eye on overall stress. Speed work and strength training are non-negotiables, as are quality sleep and quality food intake. Our thoughts matter hugely, too. We may need to rethink some things and come up with some fresh athletic goals, define our values and find purpose. That could start with asking ourselves that profound but tricky question: why do we run in the first place?

It's satisfying to think that if we run regularly, sometimes fast, lift heavy things, sleep well, eat well and think of ourselves as badass athletes we are not just potentially going to live longer, but also better. And we'll be more alive right now, too. To paraphrase the *Ted Lasso* character Dani Rojas, running is life!

CONCLUSIONS

'Ageing is an extraordinary process whereby you become the person you always should have been.'
DAVID BOWIE

'You are only young once, but you can stay immature indefinitely.'
OGDEN NASH

'Birthdays are good for you. Statistics show that the people who have the most live the longest.'
LARRY LORENZONI

'In the end, it's not the years in your life that count. It's the life in your years.'
ATTRIBUTED TO ABRAHAM LINCOLN

'Getting old is like climbing a mountain; you get a little out of breath, but the view is much better.'
INGRID BERGMAN

'Your forties are good. Your fifties are great. Your sixties are fab. And seventy is fucking awesome!'
HELEN MIRREN

Well, I don't know about you, but I'm feeling a whole lot better about this getting old(er) lark now. Yes, there are some really annoying elements to our inevitable physiological ripening, both currently and forecasted. And while this book could potentially protect you from the Four Horsemen, it can't protect you from getting run over if you're on your phone as you cross the street, or from a random lightning strike. Sorry about that.

Some of the science we look to is based on previous generations and sedentary folks and there are some truly kick-ass mature athletes all around us doing extraordinary things. We can't let chronological age be an excuse for a suboptimal life.

I find that the more I invest time into my running and my health, the more fulfilled I feel and I'm hopefully a better-rounded, more satisfied person. Which hopefully means I'm more positive, engaged and in the moment with those closest to me, and more productive in other roles, too.

Investing in our healthspan can feel selfish sometimes, but it's also an investment in all those around us. Better athlete = better health = better person.

To be the best runner we can be, firstly, we mustn't stop! We must continue being consistent, which above all means avoiding injury. We can do this by being sensible with training, maybe doing a little less, following a structure but a flexible one, with deliberate recovery, ample quality sleep and ample quality food. We need to be purposeful with sleep, prioritising it. And deliberate with our diets, being conscious of protein intake and with adequate energy overall. We must run fast. Frequently. And we must lift heavy things. Regularly.

Our mindset is so important, too. We may need some new goals and reminders of why we love this stuff in the first place. If we think of ourselves as decrepit, slow, old things, we will be. If we think of ourselves as ageless aces, we can be.

Happy midlife running!

PERSONAL REFLECTIONS

Through researching this book, I realised I was semi-accidentally doing a lot of things right. I'm lucky to have been coached by David Roche for the last five years and he has me prioritising top-end speed work and, despite my protestations, gradually reducing my volume, switching sometimes for cross-training (and sauna time). Touch wood, I've been uninjured for several years, which may be the biggest contributor towards still being competitive in ultramarathon running. It may come, but I've never had more than a couple of weeks off running. As well as sensible training, I've also been pre-emptively seeing a sports therapist, Bathford's Matt Holmes, for ten years. Usually it's a quick check over and a leg massage, but he always seems to spot a quirky imbalance in my feet or hips to work on, while a massage releases tightness in areas I hadn't yet detected, extinguishing problems before they exist.

I'll admit I'm not 100% consistent with strength work, but I've been doing it on and off for ten years, some months with more zeal than others; I know its importance and always return to it. Pete Stables has really freshened things up for me lately and I've genuinely grown (pun unintended) to enjoy it.

I've also shed that youthful idea that I must stick to the training plan, must do every run and every mile of every run. I have occasionally shortened a run, turned a workout into an easy run or taken a day off when something didn't feel quite right, physically, hormonally or just instinctively. I eat well (all plants nowadays), am grateful of Renee McGregor's hallowed advice on nutrition and haven't touched alcohol for over eighteen months. I could do better with sleep, but finally finishing this book will help.

Perhaps above all, I'm just grateful I've never lost my joy and passion for long bimbles in lumpy places. And I aim to keep it that way. There are just so many ouchy adventures to be had out there in the hills and bogs. They don't know or care what my chronological age is.

I AM AN AGELESS ACE: THE MANIFESTO

I will not go gentle into that good night.
I am older. But I am not old.
I am a midlife maestro, a timeless Titan, an ageless ace.
I will rage against my chronological age.
I will grow older disgracefully.
I refuse to admit my best days are behind me – they are ahead of me.
I will train smarter, not harder.
I will master my Masters era.
I will never be as fast again as I am today.
I will sprint like a cheetah;
I am defiantly cheating time.
I know my age is an advantage.
I will be wise about recovery, sleep, food and friendships.
I will lift heavy things, because I am strong and powerful.
I will show people what is possible.
I will sit, and eventually lie down, one day. But not this day.
I will not go gentle into that good night;
I will rage, rage against age and the dying of the light
Because I am an ageless ace.

Signed Date

ACKNOWLEDGEMENTS

Big huge thank you to Kirsty Reade for your genius and patience, and Renee McGregor for your support, generosity and knowledge – both, incidentally, are absolutely ageless aces, banging out fuss-free ultramarathons in their fifties; and to Pete Stables for your enthusiasm, knowledge and strength plans. Big thanks also to my coach David Roche and sports therapist Matt Holmes for helping to keep me injury-free; to Jon Barton, Allie Bailey, Josie Perry, Nicky Spinks, Eoin Keith, Anna Troup, Tommy Hughes, Debbie Martin-Consani, Susie Chan, Guy Woods, Holly Stables, Tom Hutchison, Jo Pavey, Jo Moseley, Tim Laney, Alex Copping and Martin Rush; to all inspirational midlife runners kicking butt; to all the amazing people at the wonderful Vertebrate Publishing who turn my incoherent nonsense into something readable and presentable, especially Emma Lockley; to tea and nut butter in general; and to Indy and Leif for giving me purpose.

BIBLIOGRAPHY

Fast After 50, Joe Friel (VeloPress, 2023)
Fuel for Thought, Renee McGregor (Vertebrate Publishing, 2025)
Good to Go, Christie Aschwanden (Macmillan, 2020)
How Bad Do You Want It?, Matt Fitzgerald (Aurum, 2016)
How Not to Age, Michael Greger (Bluebird, 2024)
How Not to Die, Michael Greger (Pan, 2017)
Lifespan, Dr David A. Sinclair (Thorsons, 2019)
More Fuel You, Renee McGregor (Vertebrate Publishing, 2022)
Next Level, Stacy T. Sims (Rodale Books, 2022)
Not Too Late, Gwendolyn Bounds (Ballantine Books, 2025)
Play On, Jeff Bercovici (Penguin Life, 2018)
Roar, Stacy T. Sims (Rodale Books, 2024)
Smart Running, Jen and Sim Benson (Vertebrate Publishing, 2024)
Spring Chicken, Bill Gifford (Oneworld Publications, 2015)
The Body, Bill Bryson (Black Swan, 2020)
The Midlife Cyclist, Phil Cavell (Bloomsbury Sport, 2021)
The Race Against Time, Richard Askwith (Vintage, 2024)
Unbreakable, Dr Vonda Wright (Vermilion, 2025)
Why We Die, Venki Ramakrishnan (Hodder Press, 2025)

REFERENCES

PART ONE: THE BAD

1. Shen, X., Wang, C., Zhou, X. et al. (2024). 'Nonlinear dynamics of multi-omics profiles during human aging', *Nature Aging*, 4: 1619–1634. https://doi.org/10.1038/s43587-024-00692-2
2. Raleigh, V. (2024). 'What is happening to life expectancy in England?', The King's Fund, https://www.kingsfund.org.uk/insight-and-analysis/long-reads/whats-happening-life-expectancy-england, accessed 22 January 2026.
3. University of Dundee (2025). 'Breakthrough study has grave consequences for "zombie cells"', https://www.dundee.ac.uk/press-release/breakthrough-study-has-grave-consequences-zombie-cells, accessed 22 January 2026.
4. López-Otín, C., Blasco, M.A., Partridge, L. et al. (2023). 'Hallmarks of aging: An expanding universe', *Cell*, 186(2): 243–278. https://doi.org/10.1016/j.cell.2022.11.001
5. Araujo, C.G., de Souza e Silva, C.G., Laukkanen, J.A. et al. (2022). 'Successful 10-second one-legged stance performance predicts survival in middle-aged and older individuals', *British Journal of Sports Medicine*, 56: 975–980. https://doi.org/10.1136/bjsports-2021-105360
6. Xiao, T., Ghatan, S., Mooldijk, S.S. et al. (2023). 'Association of bone mineral density and dementia: The Rotterdam study', *Neurology*, 100(20): e2125–e2133. https://doi.org/10.1212/WNL.0000000000207220

PART TWO: THE GOOD

1. Chen, S., Liu, Y., Yi, Y. et al. (2025). 'Long-term impacts of heatwaves on accelerated ageing', *Nature Climate Change*, 15: 1000–1007. https://doi.org/10.1038/s41558-025-02407-w
2. Guiney, H. & Machado, L. (2013). 'Benefits of regular aerobic exercise for executive functioning in healthy populations', *Psychonomic Bulletin & Review*, 20(1): 73–86. https://doi.org/10.3758/s13423-012-0345-4
3. Creer, D.J., Romberg, C., Saksida, L.M. et al. (2010). 'Running enhances spatial pattern separation in mice', *Proceedings of the National Academy of Sciences of the United States of America*, 107(5): 2367–2372. https://doi.org/10.1073/pnas.0911725107

4. Lee, D.C., Pate, R.R., Lavie, C.J. et al. (2014). 'Leisure-time running reduces all-cause and cardiovascular mortality risk', *Journal of the American College of Cardiology*, 64(5): 472–481. https://doi.org/10.1016/j.jacc.2014.04.058
5. Lee et al. (2014). 'Leisure-time running reduces all-cause and cardiovascular mortality risk.'
6. American Academy of Neurology (2018). 'Physically fit women nearly 90 percent less likely to develop dementia', https://www.aan.com/PressRoom/Home/PressRelease/1634, accessed 22 January 2026.
7. American Academy of Neurology (2022). 'Physical fitness linked to lower risk of Alzheimer's disease', https://www.aan.com/PressRoom/Home/PressRelease/4960, accessed 22 January 2026.
8. Gutierre, R.C., Rocha, P.R., Graciani, A.L. et al. (2025). 'Tau, amyloid, iron, oligodendrocytes ferroptosis, and inflammaging in the hippocampal formation of aged rats submitted to an aerobic exercise program', *Brain Research*, 1850: 149419. https://doi.org/10.1016/j.brainres.2024.149419
9. Judd, W. (2018). 'To look and feel younger, running is the real miracle drug', Runner's World, https://www.runnersworld.com/news/a20865704/to-look-and-feel-younger-running-is-the-real-miracle-drug, accessed 22 January 2026.
10. Tanaka, H. & Seals, D.R. (2008). 'Endurance exercise performance in masters athletes: Age-associated changes and underlying physiological mechanisms', *The Journal of Physiology*, 586(1): 55–63. https://doi.org/10.1113/jphysiol.2007.141879
11. Fitzgerald, M. (2025). 'Chasing the young', Endurance Mastery, https://endurancemastery.substack.com/p/chasing-the-young, accessed 22 January 2026.
12. Lepers, R. & Stapley, P.J. (2016). 'Master athletes are extending the limits of human endurance', *Frontiers in Physiology*, 7: 613. https://doi.org/10.3389/fphys.2016.00613
13. Tanaka & Seals (2008). 'Endurance exercise performance in masters athletes: Age-associated changes and underlying physiological mechanisms.'
14. Shen, X., Wang, C., Zhou, X. et al. (2024). 'Nonlinear dynamics of multi-omics profiles during human aging', *Nature Aging*, 4: 1619–1634. https://doi.org/10.1038/s43587-024-00692-2
15. Fair, R.C. & Kaplan, E.H. (2018). 'Estimating aging effects in running events', *The Review of Economics and Statistics*, 100 (4): 704–711. https://doi.org/10.1162/REST_a_00725
16. Hjelmborg, J.v., Iachine, I., Skytthe, A. et al. (2006). 'Genetic influence on human lifespan and longevity', *Human Genetics*, 119(3): 312–321. https://doi.org/10.1007/s00439-006-0144-y
17. Chen, J., Wang, Y., Zhong, Z. et al. (2025). 'Sex differences in the association of wearable accelerometer-derived physical activity with coronary heart disease incidence and mortality', *Nature Cardiovascular Research*, 4: 1539–1549. https://doi.org/10.1038/s44161-025-00732-z
18. Foulkes, S., Hewitt, D., Skow, R. et al. (2024). 'Outrunning the grim reaper: Longevity of the first 200 sub-4 min mile male runners', *British Journal of Sports Medicine*, 58: 717–721. https://doi.org/10.1136/bjsports-2024-108386
19. Rosin, B. (2017). 'Is marathon running toxic? An observational study of cardiovascular disease prevalence and longevity in 54 male marathon runners', *The Physician and Sportsmedicine*, 45(2): 105–109. https://doi.org/10.1080/00913847.2017.1288545

20. Blackmon, C.M., Tucker, L.A., Bailey, B.W. et al. (2023). 'Time spent jogging/running and biological aging in 4458 U.S. adults: An NHANES investigation', *International Journal of Environmental Research and Public Health*, 20(19): 6872. https://doi.org/10.3390/ijerph20196872

21. Werner, C.M., Hecksteden, A., Morsch, A. et al. (2019). 'Differential effects of endurance, interval, and resistance training on telomerase activity and telomere length in a randomized, controlled study', *European Heart Journal*, 40(1): 34–46. https://doi.org/10.1093/eurheartj/ehy585

22. Tucker, L.A. (2017). 'Physical activity and telomere length in U.S. men and women: An NHANES investigation', *Preventive Medicine*, 100: 145–151. https://doi.org/10.1016/j.ypmed.2017.04.027

23. LaRocca, T.J., Seals, D.R. & Pierce, G.L. (2010). 'Leukocyte telomere length is preserved with aging in endurance exercise-trained adults and related to maximal aerobic capacity', *Mechanisms of Ageing and Development*, 131(2): 165–167. https://doi.org/10.1016/j.mad.2009.12.009

24. Gries, K.J., Raue, U., Perkins, R.K. et al. (2018). 'Cardiovascular and skeletal muscle health with lifelong exercise', *Journal of Applied Physiology*, 125(5): 1636–1645. https://doi.org/10.1152/japplphysiol.00174.2018

25. Bhuva, A.N., D'Silva, A., Torlasco, C. et al. (2020). 'Training for a first-time marathon reverses age-related aortic stiffening', *Journal of the American College of Cardiology*, 75(1): 60–71. https://doi.org/10.1016/j.jacc.2019.10.045

26. Steptoe, A., Deaton, A. & Stone, A.A. (2015). 'Subjective wellbeing, health, and ageing', *The Lancet*, 385(9968): 640– 648. https://doi.org/10.1016/S0140-6736(13)61489-0

PART THREE: THE UGLY

1. Robinson S., Edwards, H.T. & Dill, D.B. (1937). 'New records in human power', *Science*, 85(2208): 409–410. https://doi.org/10.1126/science.85.2208.409

2. Pollock, M.L, Foster, C., Knapp, D. et al. (1987). 'Effect of age and training on aerobic capacity and body composition of master athletes', *Journal of Applied Physiology*, 62(2): 725–731. https://doi.org/10.1152/jappl.1987.62.2.725

3. Friel, J. (2023). *Fast After 50* (VeloPress), 108.

4. Patil, H.R., O'Keefe, J.H., Lavie, C.J. et al. (2012). 'Cardiovascular damage resulting from chronic excessive endurance exercise', *Missouri Medicine*, 109(4): 312-321.

5. Mengelkoch, L.J., Pollock, M.L., Limacher, M.C. et al. (1997). 'Effects of age, physical training, and physical fitness on coronary heart disease risk factors in older track athletes at twenty-year follow-up', *Journal of the American Geriatrics Society*, 45(12): 1446–1453. https://doi.org/10.1111/j.1532-5415.1997.tb03194.x

6. Zilinski, J.L., Contursi, M.E., Isaacs, S.K. et al. (2015). 'Myocardial adaptations to recreational marathon training among middle-aged men', *Circulation: Cardiovascular Imaging*, 8(2): e002487. https://doi.org/10.1161/CIRCIMAGING.114.002487

7. Babcock. M.C., El-Kurd, O.B., Bagley, J.R. et al. (2024). 'Acute cardiovascular responses to the 100-mi Western States Endurance Run', *Journal of Applied Physiology*, 137(5): 1257–1266. https://doi.org/10.1152/japplphysiol.00412.2024

8. Patil et al. (2012). 'Cardiovascular damage resulting from chronic excessive endurance exercise'.
9. Wen, D., Utesch, T., Wu, J. et al. (2019). 'Effects of different protocols of high intensity interval training for VO_2max improvements in adults: A meta-analysis of randomised controlled trials', *Journal of Science and Medicine in Sport*, 22(8): 941–947. https://doi.org/10.1016/j.jsams.2019.01.013
10. Curry, E. (2025). 'The gold standard VO_2 max training method?', Science for Sport, https://www.scienceforsport.com/gold-standard-aerobic-training-method, accessed 22 January 2026.
11. Lepers, R. & Stapley, P.J. (2016), 'Master athletes are extending the limits of human endurance', *Frontiers in Physiology*, 7: 613. https://doi.org/10.3389/fphys.2016.00613
12. Tanaka, H. & Seals, D.R. (2008). 'Endurance exercise performance in masters athletes: Age-associated changes and underlying physiological mechanisms', *The Journal of Physiology*, 586(1): 55–63. https://doi.org/10.1113/jphysiol.2007.141879
13. Douglas, S. (2025). 'Everything you need to know about running economy', Runner's World, https://www.runnersworld.com/training/a64150769/what-is-running-economy, accessed 22 January 2026.
14. Skovgaard, C., Christiansen, D., Christensen, P.M. et al. (2018). 'Effect of speed endurance training and reduced training volume on running economy and single muscle fiber adaptations in trained runners', *Physiological Reports*, 6(3): e13601. https://doi.org/10.14814/phy2.13601
15. Murr, S. & Pierce, B. (2019). 'How aging impacts runners' goals of lifelong running', *Physical Activity and Health*, 3(1): 71–81. https://doi.org/10.5334/paah.42
16. Mutton, D.L., Loy, S.F., Rogers, D.M. et al. (1993). 'Effect of run vs combined cycle/run training on VO2max and running performance', *Medicine and Science in Sports and Exercise*, 25(12): 1393–1397.
17. Marcell, T.J., Hawkins, S.A. & Wiswell, R.A. (2014). 'Leg strength declines with advancing age despite habitual endurance exercise in active older adults', *Journal of Strength and Conditioning Research*, 28(2): 504–513. https://doi.org/10.1519/JSC.0b013e3182a952cc
18. Lauersen, J.B., Andersen, T.E. & Andersen, L.B. (2018). 'Strength training as superior, dose-dependent and safe prevention of acute and overuse sports injuries: A systematic review, qualitative analysis and meta-analysis', *British Journal of Sports Medicine*, 52(24): 1557–1563. https://doi.org/10.1136/bjsports-2018-099078
19. Capel-Alcaraz, A.M., García-López, H., Castro-Sánchez, A.M. et al. (2023). 'The efficacy of strength exercises for reducing the symptoms of menopause: A systematic review', *Journal of Clinical Medicine*, 12(2): 548. https://doi.org/10.3390/jcm12020548
20. Steves, C.J., Mehta, M.M., Jackson, S.H. & Spector, T.D. (2016). 'Kicking back cognitive ageing: Leg power predicts cognitive ageing after ten years in older female twins', *Gerontology*, 62(2): 138–149. https://doi.org/10.1159/000441029
21. Tucker, L.A. & Bates, C.J. (2024). 'Telomere length and biological aging: The role of strength training in 4814 US men and women', *Biology*, 13(11): 883. https://doi.org/10.3390/biology13110883
22. Taylor, D.C., Dalton, J.D., Jr, Seaber, A.V. & Garrett, W.E., Jr, (1990). 'Viscoelastic properties of muscle-tendon units: The biomechanical effects of stretching', *American Journal of Sports Medicine*, 18(3): 300–309. https://doi.org/10.1177/036354659001800314

23. Burtscher, J., Strasser, B., Burtscher, M. & Millet, G.P. (2022). 'The impact of training on the loss of cardiorespiratory fitness in aging masters endurance athletes', *International Journal of Environmental Research and Public Health*, 19(17): 11050. https://doi.org/10.3390/ijerph191711050

24. Murr & Pierce (2019). 'How aging impacts runners' goals of lifelong running.'

25. Hutchinson, A. (2024). 'Most people get slower with age. But is that inevitable?', Outside Online, https://www.outsideonline.com/health/training-performance/sweat-science-aging-training, accessed 22 January 2026.

26. Hammond, C. (2016). 'The truth about whether you need less sleep as you get older', BBC Future, https://www.bbc.co.uk/future/article/20160516-the-truth-about-whether-you-need-less-sleep-as-you-get-older, accessed 22 January 2026.

27. Milewski, M.D., Skaggs, D.L., Bishop, G.A. et al. (2014). 'Chronic lack of sleep is associated with increased sports injuries in adolescent athletes', *Journal of Pediatric Orthopaedics*, 34(2): 129–133. https://doi.org/10.1097/BPO.0000000000000151

28. Leproult, R. & Van Cauter, E. (2011). 'Effect of 1 week of sleep restriction on testosterone levels in young healthy men', *JAMA*, 305(21): 2173–2174. https://doi.org/10.1001/jama.2011.710

29. Joglar, A. (2025). 'You need quality sleep for better performance – here's exactly what that means', Runner's World Australia & New Zealand, https://runnersworldonline.com.au/you-need-quality-sleep-for-better-performance-heres-exactly-what-that-means, accessed 22 January 2026.

30. Vitale, K., Owens, R., Hopkins, S.R. & Malhotra, A. (2019). 'Sleep hygiene for optimizing recovery in athletes: Review and recommendations', *International Journal of Sports Medicine*, 40(8): 535–543. https://doi.org/10.1055/a-0905-3103

31. Prather, A.A., Janicki-Deverts, D., Hall, M.H. & Cohen, S. (2015). 'Behaviorally assessed sleep and susceptibility to the common cold', *Sleep*, 38(9): 1353–1359. https://doi.org/10.5665/sleep.4968

32. Shokri-Kojori, E., Wang, G.J., Wiers, C.E. et al. (2018). 'β-Amyloid accumulation in the human brain after one night of sleep deprivation', *Proceedings of the National Academy of Sciences of the United States of America*, 115(17): 4483–4488. https://doi.org/10.1073/pnas.1721694115

33. Spiegel, K., Tasali, E., Penev, P. & Van Cauter, E. (2004). 'Brief communication: Sleep curtailment in healthy young men is associated with decreased leptin levels, elevated ghrelin levels, and increased hunger and appetite', *Annals of Internal Medicine*, 141(11): 846–850. https://doi.org/10.7326/0003-4819-141-11-200412070-00008

34. British Menopause Society (2025). 'Managing sleep disturbance during the menopause transition', https://thebms.org.uk/wp-content/uploads/2025/08/25-NEW-BMS-ToolsforClinicians-Managing-sleep-disturbance-AUGUST2025-A.pdf, accessed 22 January 2026.

35. Hackney, A.C. & Lane, A.R. (2018). 'Low testosterone in male endurance-trained distance runners: Impact of years in training', *Hormones*, 17(1): 137–139. https://doi.org/10.1007/s42000-018-0010-z

36. Res, P.T., Groen, B., Pennings, B. et al. (2012). 'Protein ingestion before sleep improves postexercise overnight recovery', *Medicine & Science in Sports & Exercise*, 44(8): 1560–1569. https://doi.org/10.1249/MSS.0b013e31824cc363

37. Zhu, H., Manson, J.E., Cook, N.R. et al. (2025). 'Vitamin D3 and marine ω-3 fatty acids supplementation and leukocyte telomere length: 4-year findings from the VITamin D and OmegA-3 TriaL (VITAL) randomized controlled trial', *American Journal of Clinical Nutrition*, 122(1): 39–47. https://doi.org/10.1016/j.ajcnut.2025.05.003

38. British Society of Lifestyle Medicine (2023). 'Two nutrients proven to stop your brain shrinking', https://bslm.org.uk/b-vitamins-and-omega-3-dynamic-duo-against-dementia, accessed 22 January 2026.

39. Neuroscience News (2021). 'A low Omega-3 index is just as strong a predictor of early death as smoking', https://neurosciencenews.com/omega-3-index-cvd-18801, accessed 22 January 2026.

40. Ahmad, S., Moorthy, M.V., Lee, I.M. et al. (2024). 'Mediterranean diet adherence and risk of all-cause mortality in women', *JAMA Network Open*, 7(5): e2414322. https://doi.org/10.1001/jamanetworkopen.2024.14322

41. Miyamoto, N., Ishihara, K., Oshima, T. et al. (2025). 'Collagen peptide supplementation enhances muscle-tendon stiffness and explosive strength: A 16-week randomized controlled trial', *Medicine & Science in Sports & Exercise*, 57(12):2877–2886. https://doi.org/10.1249/MSS.0000000000003814

42. Chen, M., Xu, L., Van Horn, L. et al. (2025). 'Association of eating duration less than 8 h with all-cause, cardiovascular, and cancer mortality', *Diabetes & Metabolic Syndrome*, 19(7): 103278. https://doi.org/10.1016/j.dsx.2025.103278

43. Konrad, A., Močnik, R., Nakamura, M. et al. (2021). 'The impact of a single stretching session on running performance and running economy: A scoping review', *Frontiers in Physiology*, 11: 630282. https://doi.org/10.3389/fphys.2020.630282

44. Brunt, V.E., Howard, M.J., Francisco, M.A. et al. (2016). 'Passive heat therapy improves endothelial function, arterial stiffness and blood pressure in sedentary humans', *Journal of Physiology*, 594(18): 5329–5342. https://doi.org/10.1113/JP272453

45. Scoon, G.S.M., Hopkins, W.G., Mayhew, S. & Cotter, J.D. (2007). 'Effect of post-exercise sauna bathing on the endurance performance of competitive male runners', *Journal of Science and Medicine in Sport*, 10(4): 259–262. https://doi.org/10.1016/j.jsams.2006.06.009

46. Laukkanen, T., Khan, H., Zaccardi, F. & Laukkanen, J.A. (2015). 'Association between sauna bathing and fatal cardiovascular and all-cause mortality events', *JAMA Internal Medicine*, 175(4): 542–548. https://doi.org/10.1001/jamainternmed.2014.8187

47. Strandberg, T.E., Strandberg, A., Pitkälä, K. & Benetos, A. (2018). 'Sauna bathing, health, and quality of life among octogenarian men: the Helsinki Businessmen Study', *Aging Clinical and Experimental Research*, 30(9): 1053–1057. https://doi.org/10.1007/s40520-017-0855-z

48. Adães, S. (2025). 'Sauna health benefits, explained: The latest research on heat therapy', Qualia, https://www.qualialife.com/sauna-health-benefits/ accessed 22 January 2026.

49. Beedie, C.J., Stuart, E.M., Coleman, D.A. & Foad, A.J. (2006). 'Placebo effect of caffeine on cycling performance', *Medicine and Science in Sport and Exercise*, 38(12): 2159–2164. https://doi.org/10.1249/01.mss.0000233805.56315.a9

50. Stoate, I., Wulf, G. & Lewthwaite, R. (2012). 'Enhanced expectancies improve movement efficiency in runners', *Journal of Sport Sciences*, 30(8): 815–823. https://doi.org/10.1080/02640414.2012.671533

51. Dunstan, D.W., Barr, E.L.M., Healy, G.N. et al. (2010). 'Television viewing time and mortality: The Australian Diabetes, Obesity and Lifestyle Study (AusDiab)', *Circulation*, 121(3): 384–391. https://doi.org/10.1161/CIRCULATIONAHA.109.894824

52. Gao, Y., Li, Q.Y., Finni, T. & Pesola, A.J. (2024). 'Enhanced muscle activity during interrupted sitting improves glycemic control in overweight and obese men', *Scandinavian Journal of Medicine & Science in Sports*, 34(4): e14628. https://doi.org/10.1111/sms.14628

53. Krzyzanowski B., Mullan A.F., Dorsey, E.R. et al. (2025). 'Proximity to golf courses and risk of Parkinson disease', *JAMA Network Open*, 8(5): e259198. https://doi.org/10.1001/jamanetworkopen.2025.9198

54. Fidra (2025). 'Concentrations of trifluoroacetic acid (TFA) in UK surface waters', https://fidra.org.uk/download/concentrations-of-trifluoroacetic-acid-tfa-in-uk-surface-waters, accessed 22 January 2026.

55. Yang, S., Cheng, Y., Chen, Z. et al. (2021). 'In vitro evaluation of nanoplastics using human lung epithelial cells, microarray analysis and co-culture model', *Ecotoxicology and Environmental Safety*, 226: 112837. https://doi.org/10.1016/j.ecoenv.2021.112837

56. Robson, D.(2022). 'Can you think yourself young?', Guardian, https://www.theguardian.com/science/2022/jan/02/can-you-think-yourself-young-ageing-psychology, accessed 22 January 2026.

57. Reverse Aging Revolution, 'TURN BACK THE CLOCK In 5 DAYS, A 1979 Study By A Harvard Professor | Dr Ellen Langer Interview Clips' [video], YouTube (uploaded 16 July 2022), https://www.youtube.com/watch?v=EVW2xC44Z34, accessed 22 January 2026.

58. Levy, B.R., Slade, M.D., Kunkel, S.R. & Kasl, S.V. (2002). 'Longevity increased by positive self-perceptions of aging', *Journal of Personality and Social Psychology*, 83(2): 261–270. https://doi.org/10.1037//0022-3514.83.2.261

59. Levy, B.R., Slade, M.D., Pietrzak, R.H. & Ferrucci, L. (2018). 'Positive age beliefs protect against dementia even among elders with high-risk gene', *PLoS One*, 13(2): e0191004. https://doi.org/10.1371/journal.pone.0191004

60. Weiss, D., Job, V., Mathias, M. et al. (2016). 'The end is (not) near: Aging, essentialism, and future time perspective', *Developmental Psychology*, 52(6): 996–1009. https://doi.org/10.1037/dev0000115

61. Jewett, S.P. (1973). 'Longevity and the longevity syndrome', *The Gerontologist*, 13(1): 91–99. https://doi.org/10.1093/geront/13.1.91

62. Harvard Study of Adult Development, https://www.adultdevelopmentstudy.org, accessed 22 January 2026.

63. Whisman, M.A., Gilmour, A.L. & Salinger, J.M. (2018). 'Marital satisfaction and mortality in the United States adult population', *Health Psychology*, 37(11): 1041–1044. https://doi.org/10.1037/hea0000677

64. Imatome-Yun, N.(2019). 'Why volunteering is one of the most powerful things you can do for your health', Blue Zones, https://www.bluezones.com/2019/07/why-volunteering-is-one-of-the-most-powerful-things-you-can-do-for-your-health, accessed 22 January 2026.

ABOUT THE AUTHORS

Damian Hall is a record-breaking ultrarunner who represented Great Britain aged forty and still competes in some of the world's toughest races, including the legendary Barkley Marathons, in his fifties. His attempt to break into the top ten at the 105-mile Ultra-Trail du Mont Blanc was made into an award-winning film, *Underdog*. Also in his forties, Damian set records on the Pennine Way, Paddy Buckley Round, the South West Coast Path, the Cape Wrath Trail and Wainwright's Coast to Coast. Aged forty-nine, he broke the record for the 185-mile Northern Traverse and won the Lakeland 100. He is a UK Athletics running coach, Level 2 Gym Instructor, Mountain Leader and a widely published journalist with a column in *Runner's World*. His previous books include the bestselling *In It for the Long Run* and award-nominated *We Can't Run Away From This*. The father of two is a co-founder of The Green Runners, and Into Ultra, a charity removing barriers to ultrarunning. He is a big fan of tea and midlife-crisis haircuts. **www.ultradamo.com**

Renee McGregor is a world-renowned sports dietitian with over twenty-five years' experience, specialising in athlete nutrition, REDs and hormonal health. From clinic days to mountainside support, Renee works tirelessly to ensure her clients are fuelled by science-backed strategies and her years of knowledge in the industry. Her practice and insight are supported by extensive experience of working in both clinical and performance nutrition, including with numerous athletes in Olympic, Paralympic and Commonwealth Games teams, professional football teams, English and Scottish

National Ballet and numerous runners, including the GB 24-Hour Team. Her books include *Fuel for Thought* and *More Fuel You*, and she is a *Runner's World* columnist and the star of the film *Unfiltered* by Summit Fever Media. She's also a trustee for Black Trail Runners and a kick-ass midlife ultra-marathon runner. **www.reneemcgregor.com**

Pete Stables is a strength and conditioning coach with over twenty years of experience working with athletes across a range of sports. He's also spent a fair bit of time under the bar himself, somehow managing to hit personal bests of a 250-kilogram squat, 150-kilogram bench press and 272.5-kilogram deadlift. In recent years, he's dabbled in a bit of endurance work too, clocking a 2:54 at the Pisa Marathon in 2024 – not too shabby for a reformed powerlifter who once believed anything over five reps counted as cardio. He's also taken part in events that most sensible people would politely decline – like running from London to Paris, stumbling his way through Nepal's Three Passes (yes, running again), and pacing Holly Stables in The Speed Project LALV, which is less of a race and more of a sleep-deprived, logistics-fuelled hallucination. He currently divides his time between training, quietly judging poor technique and trying very hard not to get roped into anything that involves public speaking or engaging with social media.